ROUTLEDGE LIBRARY EDITIONS:
CHILDREN AND DISABILITY

Volume 4

THE COSTS OF CARING

THE COSTS OF CARING
Families with disabled children

SALLY BALDWIN

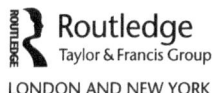

LONDON AND NEW YORK

First published in 1985 by Routledge & Kegan Paul plc

This edition first published in 2016
by Routledge
2 Park Square, Milton Park, Abingdon, Oxon OX14 4RN

and by Routledge
711 Third Avenue, New York, NY 10017

Routledge is an imprint of the Taylor & Francis Group, an informa business

© 1985 Sally Baldwin

All rights reserved. No part of this book may be reprinted or reproduced or utilised in any form or by any electronic, mechanical, or other means, now known or hereafter invented, including photocopying and recording, or in any information storage or retrieval system, without permission in writing from the publishers.

Trademark notice: Product or corporate names may be trademarks or registered trademarks, and are used only for identification and explanation without intent to infringe.

British Library Cataloguing in Publication Data
A catalogue record for this book is available from the British Library

ISBN: 978-1-138-96230-9 (Set)
ISBN: 978-1-315-64761-6 (Set) (ebk)
ISBN: 978-1-138-95103-7 (Volume 4) (hbk)
ISBN: 978-1-138-95106-8 (Volume 4) (pbk)
ISBN: 978-1-315-66840-6 (Volume 4) (ebk)

Publisher's Note
The publisher has gone to great lengths to ensure the quality of this reprint but points out that some imperfections in the original copies may be apparent.

Disclaimer
The publisher has made every effort to trace copyright holders and would welcome correspondence from those they have been unable to trace.

The publishers would like to make it clear that the views and opinions expressed, and language used in the book are the author's own and a reflection of the times in which it was published. No offence is intended in this edition.

The costs of caring

Families with disabled children

Sally Baldwin
Social Policy Research Unit
Department of Social Policy and Social Work
University of York

Routledge & Kegan Paul
London, Boston, Melbourne and Henley

For Emma

First published in 1985
by Routledge & Kegan Paul plc
14 Leicester Square, London WC2H 7PH, England
9 Park Street, Boston, Mass. 02108, USA
464 St Kilda Road, Melbourne,
Victoria 3004, Australia and
Broadway House, Newtown Road,
Henley-on-Thames, Oxon RG9 1EN, England

Set in Times 10 on 12 point
by Set Fair Limited, London
and printed in Great Britain
by The Thetford Press Limited, Thetford, Norfolk

© *Sally Baldwin 1985*

No part of this book may be reproduced in
any form without permission from the publisher,
except for the quotation of brief passages
in criticism

Library of Congress Cataloging in Publication Data

Baldwin, Sally.

The costs of caring.
(International library of social policy)
Bibliography: p.
Includes index.
1. Handicapped children—Care and treatment—
Great Britain—Costs.   2. Handicapped children—
Civil rights—Great Britain.   3. Cost and standard
of living—Great Britain.   4. Family allowances—
Great Britain.   I. Title.   II. Series.
HV888.5.B35   1985   338.4'336282   84–15022

British Library CIP data also available

ISBN 0–7100–9882–0

Contents

Acknowledgments		xi
Introduction		1
1	Financial provision for disablement in children : emergence of the policy issue	4
	The campaign for improvements in social security provision for disablement	5
	Disabled children – Thalidomide and the emergence of a social problem	8
	Thalidomide and the compensation debate	13
	Compensation, children and the law	25
2	Disabled children – rights to compensation?	32
	The argument from compassion	33
	The argument from social justice	34
	Need	35
	Rights to welfare?	36
	Disabled children – human rights to welfare	38
	Insurance rights and the redistribution of burdens	46
	Compensation rights against the state	46
	Conclusion	47
3	Measuring the costs of disablement	49
	Previous studies of the financial consequences of disability	53
4	The study – design and methods	61
	A comparison of incomes and expenditure patterns	62
	Additional information	62
	Case Studies	63
	The families with disabled children	63
	The FES control group	65
	The depth interviews	65
	The families in the study	66

vi Contents

5	Incomes	71
	Gross incomes	71
	Sources of income	72
	Earnings	72
	The work and earnings of women with disabled children	73
	The work and earnings of men with disabled children	85
	Subjective views of the child's effect on men's working lives	86
	Comparative data	89
	Income from social security	94
	The overall effect on incomes	99
	Summary	105
6	Expenditure	107
	Comparisons with the FES control	108
	Food	109
	Fuel	112
	Clothing and shoes	115
	Transport	118
	Alcohol	122
	Tobacco	123
	Durable household goods	124
	Services	125
	Housing costs	126
	Other and miscellaneous goods	127
	Adding up the costs	128
	Less regular expenditure	132
	Summary	139
7	The overall effect – ways of coping and expectations of help	141
	Strategies for coping	141
	Parents' views of the child's effect on their living standards	150
	The help that should be given to families with disabled children	154

| 8 | Conclusion | 165 |

An expenses benefit   171
An earnings-replacement benefit   172
A compensatory benefit   173
Conclusion   173

Appendix 1 Research methodology   175

Appendix 2 Case study : Andrew Cole   184

Notes and references   191

Index   207

Tables and figures

Tables

4.1	Response of families with disabled children	64
4.2	Occupation group structure	67
5.1	Gross incomes	71
5.2	Sources of income	72
5.3	Characteristics of women's paid employment	75
5.4	Reasons why paid employment was not possible	81
5.5	Men's paid employment	91
5.6	Disability benefits received	96
5.7	Benefits received and their value	97
5.8	Family income by benefits received	98
5.9	Disposable incomes relative to need	103
5.10	Real disposable incomes	104
6.1	Amount spent on food	110
6.2	Amount spent on fuel	113
6.3	Amount spent on children's clothing	116
6.4	Amount spent on transport	119
6.5	Amount spent on alcohol	123
6.6	Amount spent on tobacco	123
6.7	Amount spent on durable household goods	124
6.8	Amount spent on services	125
6.9	Amount spent on housing	126
6.10	Amount spent on other and miscellaneous goods	127
6.11	Average weekly expenditure on all commodities by families with disposable incomes of £70–£100 a week	129
6.12	Total extra cost of disablement at different income levels	132
7.1	Changes in the ways in which money is handled	144
7.2	Signs of financial stress in the preceding year	148
7.3	Parents' views of why the government should give financial help to families with disabled children	156
7.4	The type of help that parents would find most useful at present	160
A.1	Relationship of FES occupation groups to the	

	Registrar-General's classes	180
A.2	Social class distribution – based on head of household's occupation as recorded in the survey	180
A.3	Weights and weighted normal weekly earnings of men with a disabled child	182
A.4	Diseases and disorders of the children in the study	183

Figure

5.1	Median and interquartile range of gross family income by family type	100

Acknowledgments

The completion of this book, and of the study on which it was based, has depended on the assistance of a large number of people. It is very satisfying to acknowledge their help and to thank them.

In the DHSS, the encouragement of Brian McGinnis in the early stages of the study was particularly appreciated, as was his continuing interest in it subsequently.

Professor Graham Kalton, Bob Barnes of the Office of Population Censuses and Surveys (OPCS) and W. F. F. Kemsley all gave advice on sampling problems. Their assistance in helping us to make difficult decisions was invaluable, though responsibility for those decisions rests with the author.

Fieldwork for the study was carried out by Social and Community Planning Research Ltd (SCPR). Thanks are due to SCPR for executing this taxing project with such efficiency – particularly to Douglas Wood and Anne Palmer who supervised the fieldwork and coding operations. Replicating the Family Expenditure Survey (FES) was made easier by the help and advice given by the Social Survey Divison of OPCS. Their willingness to allow us access to FES procedures, from interviewer-training through to coding, made it possible to be confident that in essentials those procedures had been followed. In the Department of Employment, Ann Barber and Vic Maitland were unfailingly helpful in answering questions on FES definitions and in extracting information from the 1978 FES. Depth interviews with families with disabled children were conducted by Pauline Ashley, Rosalind Gray and Sandra Shorter whose tact, sensitivity and perceptiveness were greatly appreciated.

The help and support of my colleagues in the Social Policy Research Unit has been important throughout. Dot Lawton devised the method of drawing the sample of disabled children and monitoring response; Jane Weale undertook the preparation of the data with her usual meticulousness; Christine Godfrey made a major contribution to the analysis. It is quite literally the case that without the collaboration of these three colleagues this book could not have been written. Albert Weale made a significant contribution to Chapter 2. Jonathan Bradshaw and Kathleen Jones read and commented on an earlier version of the manuscript. The final version was typed by Su Wompra with her customary speed and accuracy.

A large debt of gratitude is owed to David Piachaud, not only for his advice on technical problems but for his unwavering belief in the study's value and in the importance of communicating the findings to a wider audience. The support and forbearance of Joe Callan in the long period while this book was being written (and not being written) is also gratefully recognised. Special thanks go to my daughter Emma who accepted the loss of my company in that time with great understanding and patience. My very particular thanks go to the friends who looked after her so well in my absence – particularly Dot Lawton, Christine Richardson and Ann and Mark Gladwin.

Finally, and most importantly, thanks are due to the families with disabled children who took part in the study. In spite of heavy demands on their time they devoted many hours to answering questions and keeping expenditure diaries. I hope that this book accurately reflects their experience and that it has some influence on the future development of policies for disabled children and their families.

Introduction

The birth of a child who is severely disabled is likely to have profound and far-reaching consequences for families. The consequences may be psychological. The stress involved in adapting to the child's condition and its long-term implications can be considerable – and may be compounded in battling for support from a confusing and often unhelpful array of 'helping' agencies. They may also be practical and physical. Severe disablement in a child will usually mean that the dependency of infancy is greatly prolonged. Hence there will be continuing demands on parents' time and energy: feeding, washing and dressing children who are unable to do these things for themselves; coping continuously with incontinence; lifting and carrying children who cannot move independently; stimulating children whose intellectual development is slow or who suffer sensory impairments; containing the behaviour of hyperactive or destructive children. These demands which tend to increase rather than diminish as children grow up, may have financial implications. Parents' earning capacity may suffer. Simultaneously the child's condition may create needs for extra or special expenditure of various sorts.

This book is primarily concerned with these financial consequences. This does not mean that the effect of a child's disablement on families' living standards is assumed to be its most important effect. The assumption is rather that if disablement does create financial stress this will compound the day-to-day problems of caring for the child and for other family members. So it is important to establish the extent to which families do suffer financially in caring for children with disabilities and to consider whether the financial support they receive at present is adequate.

A major part of this book is devoted to reporting the findings of an empirical study whose principal objective was to establish whether severe disablement in a child does affect families' incomes and expenditure patterns and, if so, to quantify the effect. This was a large-scale comparative study commissioned by the Department of Health and Social Security to inform the development of provision for disabled children and their families. We did this not only by investigating the financial impact of disablement and relating this to a number of different policy options but also by attempting to clarify the nature of collective responsibility towards disabled children and their families.

In the introductory chapters the study is set in the context of the policy debate from which it originated. Chapter 1 discusses the emergence of financial provision for disabled children as a policy issue of some importance in the early 1970s. This is linked to the general debate on financial provision for disablement which had developed in the mid-1960s and, more directly, to the Thalidomide crisis of 1971. Both were influential factors in the decision to establish a Royal Commission on Compensation for Personal Injury in 1971, part of whose remit was to clarify the respective roles of the legal and social security systems in providing financial support for disablement.

In the case of children, unlike that of adults, the Pearson Commission's view was that the origin of the condition should play no part in deciding the level of support or who should provide it. Responsibility for financial support should rest primarily with the social security system and, together with services in kind, should be substantially improved. However the reasons why society *should* provide generous financial support to disabled children and their families were not discussed by the Pearson Commission. The nature of collective responsibility for disablement in children is therefore discussed in some detail in Chapter 2.

The appropriate level of financial support will depend, in part, on the extent to which families are penalized financially by the condition, hence this study's concern to measure the financial impact of severe disablement in a child. The methodological problems of doing so are discussed in Chapter 3. Chapter 4 describes the design adopted for the study together with questions of sampling, response and the characteristics of the disabled children whose families took part.

The effect of the disabled child's condition on families' incomes is discussed in Chapter 5 and its effect on their expenditure patterns in Chapter 6, both chapters drawing extensively on comparative data from a control group of families without disabled children. Since the information on which these chapters are based is available elsewhere, technical details have been kept to a minimum.[1] It remains true that they essentially present the study's empirical findings in some detail. The justification for doing so at such length is that comparative data – particularly in relation to expenditure – have not previously been available. Their value in enabling the financial costs of caring for severely disabled children to be assessed objectively is considerable.

The combined effect of income losses and extra costs is described in Chapter 7, where information from parents themselves is used to explore how families coped with the financial constraints imposed by the child's condition and to explore their views of the help they needed or expected, from statutory agencies and from society at large. The final chapter discusses the policy implications of the present study and makes a number of recommendations for policy development, both in the short and in the longer term.

This book's main concern is with disabled children and their families. However it also has relevance for the wider issue of care for dependent people. At present 'community care' policies increasingly envisage the care of elderly and mentally handicapped people being provided outside institutions. Responsibility for their care will often fall on relatives and friends. Yet so far there has been little systematic inquiry into the costs borne by informal carers – either financial or psychological. I hope this book will stimulate both further investigation of these costs and questioning of the morality of leaving them, to such a large extent, unshared.

1 Financial provision for disablement in children : emergence of the policy issue

In 1974, following a review of social security provision for chronically sick and disabled people, the government of the day published its recommendations in a House of Commons paper.[1] No specific proposals were made in that paper for children with disabilities, though it was acknowledged that severe disablement in a child might have far-reaching effects on families' finances.[2] Instead, commitment was given to a government-funded programme of research on disablement in children.[3]

The implication was that this research would be used to inform the future development of social security provision for disabled children and their families and, in particular, of cash benefits to help redress any financial penalties created by disablement. The study whose findings are described in this book was one of the first pieces of research to be commissioned.

In the present chapter we examine how it came about that the needs of disabled children and their families had come to assume such prominence in 1974.

The first strand in the explanation lies in the fact that, from the mid-1960s onwards, financial provision for disabled people was publicly debated to a much greater extent than ever before. In this debate, although there was considerable overlap between provision for adults and for children, the needs of children came, as we shall see, to be considered separately.

A number of strands fed into the debate on social security provision for people with disabilities. One of the most important was the growth of sustained pressure on government, by people with disabilities and the organizations that represented them, for improvements in the level of cash benefits for disabled people, rationalization of these benefits into a coherent 'disability income', and an acknowledgment that both benefits and services were a matter of rights. A second was the initiation of a debate on the respective roles and responsibilities of the legal and social security systems in providing financial support for disablement. The Thalidomide crisis ensured the extension of this debate to children.

The campaign for improvements in social security provision for disablement

The key factor in triggering off this campaign was the 'rediscovery' of poverty at a time of comparative affluence for the community at large, together with research evidence that disablement was strongly associated with poverty. From the mid-1960s on, work by Abel-Smith and Townsend, Sainsbury, Harris and others[4] was influential in creating an awareness of the disabled as a group for whom existing provision was inadequate.

A second influence and locus of concern throughout the 1960s was the Labour Party. Labour was in power from 1964 to 1970. Its traditional concern with social justice, given added impetus from the American War on Poverty and Civil Rights movements, was evident in the attention paid throughout the decade to developing policy on adequate social security provision, as of right, for people with disabilities. The presence within the Labour Party of academics with considerable knowledge of both disablement and social security, such as Peter Townsend, ensured frequent and detailed discussion of the kind of social security provision for disablement which would become official party policy. The Labour Party Social Policy Committee provided a forum where party members, MPs and academics could exchange ideas and formulate policy. A wealth of documentation from that Committee reveals the breadth and detail in which proposals and options for a disability income were discussed.

In Parliament itself, the activities of a group of MPs of all parties with a strong interest in the problems of disabled people ensured that disablement was a frequent topic of discussion in the House. An All-Party Committee on Disability, formed in 1968, became an important focus for mobilizing support for legislation. It was extremely influential, for example, in creating support in 1970 for a Private Member's Bill aiming to improve dramatically the support given to disabled people by local authorities under existing legislation. The All-Party Group's lobbying resulted in Alf Morris's Chronically Sick and Disabled Persons Bill reaching the statute book quickly and without a division in either Lords or Commons.[5]

Another factor bringing disablement to prominence on the political agenda in the mid-1960s was a change in the attitudes and style brought by disabled people to their relations with government and the media. Traditionally, voluntary organizations for disabled people had been run by able-bodied people and had seen their role as providing information and welfare services for their members. They tended to co-operate with, rather than make demands on, government. The establishment of the Disablement Income Group (DIG), in 1966, was the harbinger of a change in that mode of operation. DIG was founded by Megan du Boisson and Berit Thornberry, both themselves disabled, with the explicit aim of creating pressure on government to achieve a set of specific demands in the field of social security for disabled people: 'to secure the provision for *all* disabled people of a national disability income *and* an allowance for the extra expenses of disablement.'[6] DIG was unique in that its organizers, in addition to being disabled, were educated, articulate and willing to devote time to understanding the complexities of the administrative and parliamentary systems and of the social security system itself. Their style of campaigning resembled that of pressure groups like the Child Poverty Action Group – not least in the extent to which they used information from disabled people themselves in their lobbying activities – and they addressed themselves with great energy to Parliament, to ministers, to civil servants and to the press. They were, in consequence, taken seriously in government and became influential both in helping to shape policy and in refusing to allow the interest of policy makers in the disabled to flag.

It is difficult to establish the relative importance of pressure groups and other influential interest groups in bringing about specific pieces of legislation. Whatever their respective roles in the matter, provision for disabled people assumed a high priority on the agenda of both major parties in this period – a priority mirrored and frequently serviced by activity within DHSS itself.[7]

The result was a spate of legislation[8] which, by 1971, had significantly altered the pattern of social security provision for disabled people. This was followed by a commitment, in the 1973 Social Security Act, to a fundamental review of social security provision for the chronically sick and disabled,[9] concentrating particularly on those whom the contribution-based national insurance scheme did not cover – most of whom faced, in consequence, a lifetime of dependence on means-tested supplementary benefit.

The first major new development in benefits for the disabled before 1973 had been the attendance allowance, whose novelty lay in its being the first benefit outside the industrial injuries and war pensions schemes to help with the costs of disablement rather than replacing earnings. The attendance allowance had originally been tacked on to Richard Crossman's 1969 proposals to reform the retirement pensions scheme,[10] lost when the Labour government lost the 1970 election. The degree of consensus in Parliament on the urgency of increasing help for the disabled is indicated by the speed with which the proposal for an attendance allowance was retrieved from the politically contentious pensions proposals and enacted by the incoming Conservative government in 1970.[11]

The attendance allowance is discussed in detail below.[12] However one important consequence of the discussions within the DHSS that preceded the decision to make attendance needs the criterion for a new benefit was the decision to undertake, through the Office of Population Censuses and Surveys (OPCS), the first ever representative survey of disabled people in the United Kingdom. One of this survey's purposes was to provide estimates of the numbers of people likely to be eligible for the new benefit. There had never been a sample survey of the disabled population, hence the size of the eligible population, the take-up and the cost of the proposed benefit could not be assessed. In 1969, therefore, Amelia Harris's study, which provided not only estimates of prevalence but highly influential information on the incomes and standards of living of disabled people, took place.[13]

Children were not included in this exercise. As a study by Bradshaw makes clear, children were not a group among the disabled who had received much attention in the discussions of disability that took place from the mid-1960s on.[14] Having made an extensive search of government and academic papers, parliamentary debates, the literature of political parties and of voluntary organizations and pressure groups concerned with the disabled, Bradshaw found no evidence that disabled children were in the forefront of anyone's mind in the 1960s. They were an invisible group whose needs were assumed to be met by existing services,[15] though there were of course many individuals within the DHSS and elsewhere who were familiar with the problems experienced by disabled children and their families. Given, however, the general lack of awareness in government or within the DHSS that severe disablement in children created burdens which were largely untouched by existing services, it is not surprising that children under sixteen were excluded from the Harris survey.[16]

With hindsight, the decision to exclude children was unfortunate. By the time the DHSS had concluded the review of social security provision promised in the 1973 Social Security Act, on which the 1974 House of Commons Paper was based, disabled children and public response to their families' problems had become a highly charged issue, much discussed in Parliament and the media. The 1974 House of Commons Paper accepted that severe disablement in a child might have far-reaching economic, practical and psychological consequences for families and that there were gaps both in services and in cash benefits for this group. However the absence of reliable information, resulting from children's exclusion from the 1969 survey, made it impossible to plan the appropriate development of support. 'Where disabled children are concerned, we lack adequate information about their numbers and about the precise character of their needs.'[17] Hence the commitment to research.

But how did disabled children, previously notable by their absence from policy discussions of disablement in the 1960s and early 1970s, suddenly come to be identified in this government document as a problem group about whom more needed to be known?

Disabled children – Thalidomide and the emergence of a social problem

The way in which problems, or problem groups, surface are defined as the legitimate object of social policy and come to be given priority by governments is a staple concern of students of social policy and one which has been examined both in the abstract and in relation to specific policy developments.[18] The major work on social policy development in Britain, by Hall *et al.*,[19] represents an attempt to move beyond the simplistic thesis that when needs come to light, public feeling is stirred and government responds to that feeling by allocating resources. Governments do not, according to Hall *et al.*, commit resources on a large scale to a previously undefined problem group simply in response to a wave of strong public feeling. Many other forces and factors are involved in the policy-making process, and the priority that any issue ultimately attains will relate to how it is assessed in relation to three criteria: its legitimacy, the feasibility of doing something to help, and the support the government can command for a proposed initiative.

Bradshaw has analysed the process by which, in 1973, resources were suddenly allocated, via the Family Fund, to severely disabled children – a group which, as we have seen, had attracted practically no attention before that time. He poses the question 'Why did the needs of families with handicapped children gain precedence over other needs in November 1972, and why and how was the Family Fund established to meet those needs?'[20] Though establishing a degree of congruence between the origins of the Family Fund and the particular form it took and Hall *et al.*'s explanatory framework, Bradshaw's analysis extends that framework by establishing that there *are* policy developments in which 'public feeling' plays a much more important part than Hall *et al.* would suggest, the Family Fund being one such development.

In fact, as he demonstrates, the *only* reason why families with disabled children suddenly became visible to government and were acknowledged to be bearing unacceptably heavy burdens was the public response to the Thalidomide affair, and the pressure placed on government to direct help quickly to families with Thalidomide-damaged children.

The Thalidomide affair has been described at length elsewhere.[21] The salient facts can be summarized as follows. As a result of taking the drug Thalidomide in early pregnancy, some 400 women in the United Kingdom gave birth, between 1959 and 1962, to children with gross congenital abnormalities. The drug, which was withdrawn in November 1961, was produced and marketed in the United Kingdom by Distillers Company (Biochemicals) Limited. In the decade after it had been identified as causing deformities, the parents of the deformed children struggled, unsuccessfully, to obtain adequate compensation from Distillers through the legal system. Public discussion of their dealings with Distillers was stifled by the *sub-judice* rule which limited press coverage to simply reporting their attempts to achieve a satisfactory settlement. However, in September 1972 the *Sunday Times*, which had been following the legal struggles of the families since 1967, decided to risk prosecution for contempt by publishing the first of a series of articles called 'Our Thalidomide Children: A Cause for National Shame'. As Bradshaw says:

These articles led to a massive upsurge of public concern about Thalidomide children which involved the courts, Parliament, the government, shareholders, the rest of the press, trade unions, local authorities, the large city institutions, retailers, consumers, and many other organizations, institutions and individuals.[22]

The government initially tried to present the matter as not their concern, but a matter for the courts to decide. Finally, however, they were forced to act, setting up the Family Fund which would, in the interim, provide help with needs not within the province of the statutory authorities.

For the Thalidomide children themselves, the direct results of this upsurge of public feeling included a vast improvement in the compensation offered by Distillers and the help provided by the Family Fund. However, the Thalidomide affair also raised issues and led to developments which went far beyond the immediate situation of the 400 or so Thalidomide-damaged children. Two important and related consequences which have a bearing on the DHSS decision to sponsor a research programme, and on the focus of the study reported here, are discussed below.

The first was that public and parliamentary attention came to be focussed, not only on Thalidomide-damaged children, but on all severely disabled children, whatever the origin of their condition. This widening of the discussion to include other severely disabled children was fairly predictable. Parliamentary and media coverage of the plight of the Thalidomide families and the paucity of the help they had received from the statutory services prompted responses from parents, voluntary organizations and professions concerned with other types of disability which indicated that the problems experienced by the Thalidomide families were not unique to them but shared by many other families with disabled children.

Though public awareness of them was almost non-existent the difficulties of these families had, nevertheless, to be coped with. One of the few studies of the effect of a child's disablement on family life, the report of a working party chaired by Dame Eileen Younghusband,[23] had invited submissions from parents of severely disabled children. These provided evidence of the volume of frustration and misery waiting to pour through the breach created by the public discussion of the Thalidomide families' problems.

The general picture which formed in the wake of the Thalidomide crisis was that the failure of existing policies, where disablement in children was concerned, was general rather than specific to the victims of Thalidomide.

From the government's point of view it was almost impossible to respond to the Thalidomide children without at the same time doing something for other severely disabled children. This was partly because it would, rightly, have been attacked as inequitable. It was also because a way had to be found of giving help to the Thalidomide children, and hence avoiding further public censure, without appearing to interfere in the legal dispute between Distillers and the Thalidomide families. Giving help to them, not as a unique group, but within a scheme offering help to *all* severely disabled children was one way of resolving these difficulties. In creating the Family Fund the government, in effect, made a formal declaration that, since severe disablement in children had been found to be inadequately supported by existing policies, more help would be made available to their families as a matter of urgency:

> The Government must recognise that there are others born with desperate congenital disabilities which gravely burden their families and which are as severe as the loss of limbs due to Thalidomide. Such families are inevitably involved in all manner of special needs. Many of these needs are the responsibility of statutory authorities, but there are other forms of help outside these responsibilities which could improve the life of a child and reduce the burden on its family. The Government accept that more needs to be done for children with very severe congenital disability, whether or not caused by the taking of Thalidomide. . . . The Government have therefore decided to make the sum of £3 million available for this purpose, virtually at once. It is not intended that this money should be by way of compensation for being disabled, but rather that it should serve to complement the services already being provided by statutory and voluntary bodies to help the families concerned.[24]

It had originally been intended to restrict the Family Fund's coverage to children with very severe congenital Thalidomide-like deformities. Sir Keith Joseph, announcing the Fund's creation and whom it would help, said:

> I must emphasize that I am talking about children congenitally

disabled – and by that I mean children with very severe congenital disabilities found to be present at birth or immediately after. What we have in mind are children suffering from the most severe conditions analogous to the lack of limbs, such as those suffering from the extremely damaging forms of, for instance, spina bifida.[25]

In fact it proved impossible so to limit the Fund's coverage. By the time its working guidelines were being drawn up it had become clear that a much wider range of handicaps, including mental handicap, blindness and deafness, must be included. Two years after the Fund had begun to operate, the requirement that the disability be present 'at birth or immediately after' was dropped.

The Thalidomide affair, then, and the government's action in setting up the Family Fund served to define and to institutionalize severe disablement in children as a social policy problem whose parameters the government was committed to delineating through research.

The subsequent experience of the Family Fund in responding daily to families' expressed practical needs consolidated this process – not least because of the close communication that existed between the Fund's administrators and the DHSS.

The period since the Fund's inception has seen a burgeoning of activity on disablement in children, much of it testifying to the fact that the topic is one which still has the power to spark off public debate. There has been a Royal Commission on Civil Liability and Compensation for Personal Injury;[26] discussion and legislation on the state's responsibility for vaccine-damaged children;[27] legislation on the right of children disabled before birth to sue for damages;[28] Committees of Enquiry into the child health and education services;[29] and, at the other end of the scale, the mounting of a number of research projects investigating how individual families can be helped to manage their child's condition.[30] More recently, in the course of 1981, children with disabilities were again a source of public debate and controversy. The issue in this case was whether infants known to be severely disabled at birth could legitimately (and legally) be allowed to die and who should be involved in such decisions.[31]

Scandals and crises are often deplored as blood-letting rituals which allow the public to express indignation, find a scapegoat and quickly forget the real problems. In the case of severely disabled children this may be less true – perhaps because the issues raised in the wake of the Thalidomide debate are so difficult and so compelling.

Thalidomide and the compensation debate

Another important consequence of the Thalidomide affair was the extension, explicitly to children, of the debate already in progress, on the appropriate roles of the legal and social security systems in providing compensation for disablement – the second strand in the debate on financial provision for disablement identified above.

Concern with financial provision for people incapacitated by sudden accident or injury, or by disease, was neither new nor confined to the United Kingdom when the Thalidomide crisis occurred. This concern reflected the growing awareness, already described, of the association between disablement and poverty. More specifically, it reflected growing knowledge of the circumstances of different groups of disabled people and the way these depended on what were characterized as arbitrary and irrational criteria for financial support from a number of different systems. In this period the lack of coherence in the system of financial support for disabled people came increasingly under scrutiny from academics and pressure groups alike.

One cause of this critical scrutiny was the fact that in most industrialized societies three parallel systems had developed to provide financial help for people whose earnings were interrupted by disability. Typically the two most important sources of help were the legal system of compensation and a collectively-funded social security system. Private insurance was a third, though much less important, source. By the mid-1960s in many countries the continuing expansion of the social security system, and the drive to improve its provisions, made the anomalies, overlaps and gaps created by the interaction of the legal and social security systems more obvious and, increasingly, more criticized. Growing awareness that the legal system was in fact funded by the community at large made criticisms of the way it allocated benefits seem more legitimate. Scrutiny revealed that it was extremely expensive to administer and allocate benefits with no regard to socially determined priorities. This led to a widespread questioning of the continuing role of the legal system in financial provision for disablement.[32] It also led to the much more difficult search for acceptable alternatives within the social security system. As the Woodhouse Commission on Compensation in New Zealand reported in 1967: 'The Common Law remedy has performed a useful function in the past, but it has been increasingly unable to grapple with the present needs of society, and something better should be found.'[33]

Atiyah, in an authoritative study of compensation in Britain, made the same point

> Widespread dissatisfaction with the tort system as a method of compensating people for personal injuries has become apparent throughout the entire common law world, not to mention Scandinavia and other countries with different legal systems and traditions. The result has been a stream of proposals for reform, but though there is now virtual unanimity in condemning the existing tort system, there is much less agreement about what to put in its place.[34]

Two facts made it inevitable that the relationship between the legal system of compensation for personal injury and social security provision *would* ultimately be questioned. First, collective provision for disablement arose primarily because the legal system was inadequate for dealing with the majority of cases in which accident or injury interrupted earnings. It was seen in the nineteenth century to be inefficient and unsuitable and has not changed significantly since then.[35] Second, as the social security system has grown it has come to embody assumptions and goals which conflict at a basic level with those of the legal system. For both these reasons it was inevitable that questions would eventually be raised as to whether the resources consumed in distributing benefits to a minority through the tort system might not be more appropriately distributed, on more rational and equitable principles, through the social security system. At that point the residual role of the tort system was also bound to be questioned. Such questioning would, of course, reveal tensions between, on the one hand, those with a vested interest in maintaining the tort apparatus (principally the legal profession and trades unions) and those pressing for reform and rationalization.

In the United Kingdom these underlying tensions surfaced when a Royal Commission on Civil Liability and Compensation for Personal Injury was set up in 1972 under the chairmanship of Lord Pearson. There were two triggers for the establishment of the

Pearson Commission, neither, as Walker and Townsend point out,[36] related to pressure for improvements in the system of benefits for disabled people. The first was the Robens Committee on Health and Safety at Work's recommendation that an enquiry to set up into the basis of paying compensation for injuries at work.[37] The second was concern over the (non)payment of compensation to children damaged by Thalidomide.[38]

Beyond these direct antecedents, however, the setting up of the Royal Commission reflected the pervasiveness of concern both about the legal system of compensation itself and about financial provision for disablement in general. The time was ripe for a rigorous analysis of who should provide what for disablement and why – with the principles implicit in both legal and social security systems coming equally under scrutiny. This could, and should, have been the task the Pearson Commission set itself.

In the event, most commentators agree that the Pearson Commission avoided these important but difficult questions, settling instead for a very limited interpretation of its terms of reference.[39] Thus, in the case of disabled children, its deliberations tended to focus mainly on practical matters such as families' needs and problems rather than the more fundamental questions: what was meant by compensation, for example, and why should families with disabled children be compensated at all; what form should compensation take – that is, what mix of cash and services was appropriate; what was compensation *for*, and who should be compensated – the child or the family; was the situation of disabled children special and best dealt with through social security and service provision designed for families and children, or could their needs be met better through systems largely designed with disablement as the common denominator and, as often as not, the disabled adult as the presumed target?

Questions like these had not been raised in the public discussions of compensation provoked by the Thalidomide crisis, where the discussion focused predominantly on families' pressing needs and the failure of both legal and social welfare systems to assuage these. This is not surprising; the issues involved are complex and theoretical. It is surprising, however, that they were ignored to such an extent by the Pearson Commission, whose recommendations for disabled children, though generous, were based on unexamined and uncritical views of the community's responsibility towards disabled children and their families. It could be argued that one important reason for the government's subsequent failure to act on their recommendations was precisely Pearson's failure to articulate a strong and reasoned case for compensation for disabled children and their families. Compensation is discussed in the next chapter. As a basis for that discussion we look here at what is actually provided through the legal and social security systems, comparing their explicit, and occasionally implicit, objectives.

The legal system of compensation for personal injury

The earliest financial provision for disablement, the common law system of compensation for wrongs, or 'torts', caused by another person, goes back to the middle ages. 'Civil liability in tort and in delict is the oldest method of obtaining compensation for personal injury. For a long time it was the most important.'[40] Though fault or negligence has come to be the foundation of tort compensation this was not always so. As Walker and Maclean point out, the original function of tort was the limiting of individual conflict in society; blameworthiness, or fault in the person responsible was not important.

> Historically, the tort award functioned as a way of institutionalising reaction to a wrong, thereby limiting the dimensions of an individual conflict. In Scotland the express aim of the action of settlement was 'the pacifying of the rancour of the injured person', and Scottish law calls this branch of the law reparation. The amount of payment was related to the dignity of the victim rather than any actual loss suffered.[41]

It was not until the nineteenth century (largely as a result of the increasing number of traffic and industrial accidents) that the principle of negligence became firmly embedded in the law. (Negligence is 'the omission to do something which a reasonable man, guided upon those considerations which ordinarily regulate the conduct of human affairs, would do, or doing something which a prudent and reasonable man would not do.'[42]) Today it is the basis of liability in tort actions. 'Fault is like a magic talisman; once it is established, all shall be given to the injured party.'[43] The tort system awards compensation for those wrongs which can be proven to the satisfaction of the court – the burden of proof

Financial provision for disablement in children 17

resting with the plaintiff – to have arisen from the defendant's negligence. Like all complex systems tort has a multiplicity of manifest and latent functions, discussed both in the standard legal texts[44] and, more critically, by Atiyah, Ison and other academic commentators.[45] Its most important functions, however, are compensation and deterrence – the compensation of the injured individual and the prevention of similar wrongs in the future. To these has been added, more speculatively, expiating the wrongdoer's guilt and satisfying the injured individual's desire for justice:

> If a person by rash or careless conduct causes injury to another, the wrongdoer has, or ought to have, a feeling of guilt which needs to be expiated, and the victim has a feeling of indignation which needs to be appeased, and the expiation and appeasement are achieved by a payment of compensation.[46]

Here, only the compensation of the injured individual is considered.

Compensation is a word that is semantically diffuse. It has a number of meanings and they are commonly used neither precisely nor one at a time. So complex linguistic and philosophical knots have to be unravelled before questions about the ways in which the legal and social security systems overlap in providing 'compensation' can be answered. In the following section an account is given of what the tort system currently aims to do, and of how it does that – concentrating on *de facto* compensation more than on the theoretical issues. This is then contrasted with the aims and practice of the social security system.

Broadly, the tort system aims to provide full compensation to the person who has suffered injury or illness as a result of some identifiable person's negligence – to restore them fully to the position they were in before the negligent act. It does this through cash payments which invariably take the form of a lump sum.

Atiyah distinguishes three meanings of the term compensation as it is embodied in tort:[47]

> It may be granted *as an equivalent for what has been lost* – earnings, or money paid out for services, or other expenses or property lost or damaged such as a car or house.
> It may be granted *as a substitute or solace for what has been lost*. Some losses are not financial – loss of amenity, for

example, of ability to follow pastimes, of looks and so on. In these cases awards can be made to enable the victim to afford other sources of pleasure.

It may be granted *to equalise the position of an individual in relation to others*. That is, money is awarded to people to assist them to lead lives as close to those of normal people as possible.

Tort awards reflect these different meanings. Within a broad distinction between awards for pecuniary and non-pecuniary losses, they fall into three main groups: awards for income loss; expenses; and pain, suffering and 'loss of amenity'.

Loss of income This includes actual income loss since the injury, loss of future income and loss of earning capacity – that is, the risk that the plaintiff will, because of his injury, at some time in the future lose his job, even if he is not suffering any loss of earnings at the time of the hearing.

Expenses This includes all the costs incurred or likely to be incurred by the plaintiff as a result of his injury. 'These may, for example, include the cost of domestic help, nursing care or similar attendance, extra wear and tear on clothes, and the purchase of special appliances needed to cope with physical disability.'[48] It also includes the cost of 'services rendered and expenses incurred by others'[49] for the plaintiff's benefit – for example nursing care given by a relative. Finally, costs incurred in replacing services previously provided by the plaintiff are also recoverable – the cost, for example, of paying someone to undertake the tasks previously performed by an injured housewife.

Pain, suffering and loss of amenity It might seem illogical to compensate a non-pecuniary loss with money. The Pearson Commission, defending this apparent illogicality, identified three functions of awards for non-pecuniary loss:

> First, a conventional award may serve as a palliative. Pain and suffering and loss of amenity are real enough, at least for the seriously injured plaintiff; and he may well feel entitled to some reparation where these misfortunes befell him because of an injury for which someone else is liable. Secondly, an award for non-pecuniary loss may enable the plaintiff to purchase alternative sources of satisfaction to replace those he has lost. Thirdly,

it may help to meet hidden expenses caused by his injury.[50]

Pain and suffering and loss of amenity can cover a wide range of effects – from physical pain, disfigurement, discomfort and loss of enjoyment of life to 'any mental suffering caused by knowledge of . . . shortened life expectancy'.[51]

In summary, then, the tort system recognizes that disablement can result in earnings loss, expenses, opportunity costs for friends and relatives, and pain and suffering for the disabled person. It holds that all can be compensated with money and seeks to provide *full compensation*. It provides a creative, individualized compensation scheme, the scale and exact form of the compensation package being worked out for each individual – though only for the very small number of people who are injured as a result of someone else's negligence, are aware that redress can be sought through the courts, are willing to do that and able to prove fault. As a system it has no concern with need or with establishing priorities – between disabled people or for society as a whole. Though extremely expensive to administer, it accepts high administrative costs as a by-product of fully and sensitively compensating individuals while also fulfilling the social functions of deterring similar negligent acts and meeting the social need for justice to be done and seen to be done.

Social security provision for disablement

Social security provision for disablement grew out of the inadequacy of the tort system in meeting the needs of the majority of people whose earnings were interrupted by injury or illness arising from work. Industrialization, in the nineteenth century, was accompanied by industrial injury and disease on a much wider scale than previously experienced. In many cases negligence simply could not be proven. Even where it could, compensation was often not awarded by the courts because employers were protected from having damages awarded against them by what Atiyah describes as 'the three doctrinal defences which the courts had evolved for the protection of employers'.[52] These were:

> The doctrine of common employment – denying liability when the negligence was that of a fellow worker.
> The doctrine of contributory negligence – denying liability where the workman was partly responsible for his injuries.

The doctrine of *volenti non fit injuria* – denying liability for injuries occurring from a known and obvious risk.

In consequence the tort system hardly ever provided compensation to those injured in industrial accidents. The victims of such accidents were, as Atiyah says, usually left with nothing except poor or charitable relief to live on.

With the growing power of organized labour in the late nineteenth century, alternative methods of providing for industrial disablement were sought, and found. The Workmen's Compensation Act of 1897 marks the beginning of a move towards collective provision through the social security system for the financial disruption caused by industrial disablement. This Act severed the link between compensation and the need to prove negligence, establishing that any workman had a right to compensation for any accident 'arising in and out of the course of his employment'.

The period since 1897 has seen the refinement of industrial injuries legislation and the slow development of income maintenance as a right for people whose disablement does not arise from industrial causes.[53] It has also seen the growth of collective provision, through the social security system, for a wide range of contingencies in which income is lost or reduced – reaching its apogee in Beveridge's plan to provide protection for all contingencies beyond the capacity of the individual to provide for 'from the cradle to the grave'.

Fault or negligence has practically no[54] place in that system. This does not mean that social security provision for disablement has developed in a wholly logical way according to the severity of disablement and personal need. Benefits are now paid according to the origins of the disablement, reflecting both social values and a presumed need to preserve incentives. The highest benefits go to those injured in war or at work and, after that, to those with adequate national insurance contribution records. People with no, or inadequate, contribution records receive the lowest benefits.

In comparing provision for disablement in the legal and social security systems, and in attempting to establish whether they embody similar or different notions of compensation, two important points have to be borne in mind. First, the two systems have entirely different goals and operate under entirely different constraints; second, neither is completely static. Social security is still evolving and changing. In doing so it borrows ideas and principles from other parts of the social security system in this country and elsewhere, and from other systems entirely. So social security provision for disablement has, as it has expanded, been influenced by the more generous provision available to a minority in tort. The disablement pensions and special allowances that are available in the war pensions and industrial injuries schemes draw on the tort model. The fairly new non-contributory benefits to help with the special expenses of people not injured in military service or employment drew, in turn, on the industrial injuries/war pensions model. Tort for its part, though so slowly as to be almost imperceptible, has begun to show signs of influence from ideas and concepts used in the social policy field – particularly the concept of 'need'.[55]

Differences in aims, principles and methods between the two systems remain considerable. The social security system's focus is not, as it is in tort, the disabled individual, or even all disabled people, but the whole community. Its basic objective is to ensure a minimum standard of living for *all* citizens. Provision, or improved provision, for any group has to be determined in the light of the resources available: social security objectives 'are pursued within the purpose of the national economy, which seeks to maximise national income.'[56] Account has also to be taken of competition between groups for the available resources. Resource allocation within the social security system is likely to reflect the dominant social and economic values of the time. The redistribution of the community's income through the fiscal and social security systems is essentially an ideological exercise, reflecting and reinforcing those values. The disabled are only one group among many in need. Provision for them, or for different sub-groups of people with disabilities, will be influenced among other things by what is seen as necessary for economic efficiency; by the values society attaches to disablement in comparison, for example, with old age or unemployment, and by the power or influence the disabled can command as a group.

In delivering and building on the objective of minimum subsistence, the principles that are brought into play in social security reflect a concern with equity, efficiency, the establishing of priorities and the meeting of socially recognized needs. These are very different from the principles underlying tort, with its pursuit of individualized justice and full compensation, regardless of cost or need. Nor does the public accountability characteristic of decision-making in the field of social security have any parallel in tort.

All this being so, it is quite unlikely that full compensation could ever be what the social security system sought to provide.

This is not to say that compensation is not *one* function of the social security system, though it is difficult to state precisely the extent and purpose of compensatory payments or the element of compensation within different benefits. Titmuss, for example, identifies compensation as one of the functions of benefits (whether in cash or in kind) in certain circumstances, but stresses that they may simultaneously fulfil other functions. So, though some benefits function as 'compensation for identified disservices, compensation for unidentifiable disservices and compensation for unmerited handicap', they also have other functions.[57] Jones, on the other hand, sees a more limited role for compensation.

> The notion of compensation is . . . limited in scope. A compensatory right can only be a right to reparation for injury; it cannot extend to the provision of positive benefits. Moreover, it can be invoked only in so far as society generally can be held responsible for an individual's disadvantaged condition.'[58]

McClements, as an economist, uses a very different notion of compensation, while identifying it as one of the three 'primary objectives' of the social security system: 'maintaining a minimum standard of living for the population; replacing earnings; and providing compensation.'[59] He sees earnings-replacement (by which he in fact means earnings-relation in benefits) as different from compensation. Yet since both represent an attempt to restore people, more closely than minimum subsistence rates of benefit allow, to some original position, both could be seen as partial compensation.

One reason for the difficulty of establishing the extent of the compensatory principle within the social security system is semantic. The word itself is commonly used in (at least) three senses in relation to provision by the state. The first simply relates to the replacement of earnings for the duration of their loss and carries no notion of reparation for harm inflicted by others. The second carries the notion of a payment made in consequence of some unanticipated injury or loss, such as redundancy or industrial disablement. The third relates to making good disadvantage whose origins are obscure. Perhaps the only way to avoid confusion is to use the word compensation in a neutral sense, always specifying what it is *for* or why it is owed.

A second, and possibly more important, reason for difficulty in tracking down and understanding the way the social security system compensates people arises from the nature of the system and the way it has evolved. Social security provision in Britain, as in most countries, has developed not according to explicit, rational and pre-ordained goals, but pragmatically. Perhaps the strongest principle guiding its growth is a willingness to improve provision as and when this can be afforded – improvements will be made and new forms of help introduced on whatever principle can be found to suit the occasion, so long as this does not too clearly conflict with the dominant values and goals of the system as a whole. So there is an ever-present willingness to introduce an element of compensation in benefits – that is, to take them above a basic minimum. This is done by real increases in benefit rates and in earnings-relation. It can also take the form of differential benefit rates and special supplements for particular groups or contingencies – for example, the higher rates of industrial injury benefit, contributory invalidity allowances and invalidity pensions. Industrial injury and war pensions special allowances and the non-contributory 'civilian' expenses allowances represent a willingness to compensate for some of the costs of disability. Disablement benefit itself, for war pensioners and the industrially injured – compensating for both loss of faculty (and hence pain and suffering) and implicitly some loss of earnings – represents the wish both to compensate people disabled in socially valuable and necessary pursuits, and also to ensure a continued incentive to work or serve in the armed forces.

So, while the social security system does not aim for full compensation in the way the tort system does, it does match the three actual constituents of the tort award – though at different rates according to the cause of disability and its severity.

Earnings-loss is compensated at different rates – ranging from the non-contributory invalidity pensions provided at 60 per cent of contributory invalidity pension to the much more generous amounts paid in injury benefit, and through the special hardship and unemployability supplements of the war pensions and industrial injuries schemes.

Expenses are compensated in a variety of ways, again depending on cause and severity of disablement – through supplements to the industrial injuries and war pensions schemes, attendance and mobility allowances and the Family Fund. The supplementary benefits scheme, the National Health Service (Hospital Payments) Act, and the Department of Employment also provide for some of the costs arising both from disablement itself and from hospital and work costs.

Compensation in cash for non-pecuniary loss is, however, virtually absent from the social security scheme, figuring only as an element in disablement benefit and in the hospital treatment allowance supplement in the industrial injuries and war pensions schemes. Even there, as the Pearson Commission pointed out, there is some overlap between compensation for loss of amenity and for the loss of earnings consequent on loss of faculty. Financial compensation for pain and suffering is, it seems, a luxury not to be afforded within the mainstream of social security provision – especially when so many claimants receive only the basic subsistence level of benefit. The only exception to this general rule is found in the lump sum award made by the DHSS to vaccine-damaged people. To some extent, however, the services that are provided to disabled people are a form of non-pecuniary compensation for non-pecuniary losses.

This raises the point that cash payments through the social security system are only part of the compensation the state makes to disabled people. The Pearson Commission, looking for a definition of compensation that fitted with its terms of reference, concluded that compensation from many sources had to be taken cognizance of:

> Our terms of reference . . . seemed to envisage compensation as being largely confined to an award by the courts, or a settlement out of court, arising out of the liability of one person to pay damages in respect of the death or personal injury of another. We were in no doubt that the term must be given a wider meaning.
>
> We define compensation for personal injury as the provision of something to the injured person (or to his dependents if he has been killed) in consequence of the injury and for the purpose of removing or alleviating its ill effects. . . . We are directly concerned only with monetary or cash compensation, but in considering how much money is required we must take

account of compensation provided in other ways.[60]

Dominant among these 'other ways' were the cash and services provided through the social welfare system.

Services include the medical and other services provided free of charge or at low cost by the National Health Service and by local authority social services departments. Services may also include help towards rehabilitation, domestic help and travel facilities. Goods may include such things as wheelchairs, walking aids, special clothing or special equipment. Real property may include a suitable dwelling or adaptation of an existing dwelling. All these diminish the need for cash compensation. If they had to be paid for, more money would be required.[61]

Services, then, can compensate people with disabilities – largely fulfilling what Atiyah saw as the third function of cash payments in tort – that is, equalizing the position of the disabled person in relation to his peers and restoring him physically, emotionally and socially, as far as possible, to normality.

So, through the social security system and the welfare state generally, the types of compensation offered to a few in tort, are matched for the mass of disabled people. The match is, however, in the type rather than the degree of compensation. The disabled have to compete with other groups. Their status is low. Improvements depend heavily on prevailing ideologies, the state of the economy and sustained pressure on government. Tort benefits a very small minority and is expensive to administer, but serves as an ideal model of provision on which, when resources permit, the social security system can draw.

In the following section the way each of these systems provide for children with disabilities is outlined.

Compensation, children and the law

The damage caused by Thalidomide, and the difficulties experienced in claiming compensation from the manufacturers of the drug, led, as we have seen, to the question of compensation for Thalidomide-damaged children being specifically included in the Pearson Commission's terms of reference. Thalidomide itself had affected only some 400 children in the United Kingdom. However the issue of compensation arose in two other connections while the

Pearson Comission was sitting: first in relation to children damaged *in utero* and second in relation to children allegedly disabled as a result of vaccination. In both cases legislation was eventually passed which allowed such children to claim compensation. In the case of children damaged *in utero* the Congenital Disabilities (Civil Liability) Act 1976 established their right to sue for damages at common law. In the case of vaccine damage the Vaccine Damage Payments Act 1979 enabled lump-sum compensatory payments to be claimed from DHSS where it could be established that vaccination had caused severe disability. Both issues created considerable public discussion. In addition, as noted earlier, the needs of disabled children featured prominently in major reports on the child health services and on education for children with special needs. On the social security front attention was drawn to gaps in the coverage of benefits for disabled children by the much publicized case of Jimmy Martin, a limbless boy repeatedly refused an attendance allowance at either higher or lower rate. Finally, while the Commission was sitting, the Family Fund came into being and began to amass evidence on the circumstances of families with disabled children, much of which was communicated directly to the Commission by the Family Fund research team.

The issue of disablement in children must, therefore, have been very much in the forefront of the Commission's minds. Their deliberations on disablement in children and the form support or compensation for them should take are extremely interesting.

As the Pearson Commission discovered, the legal system can provide compensation for only a tiny minority of disabled children. The proportion of children disabled by accident or illness after birth is only 10 per cent of the total number of severely disabled children, and relatively few of these can, or wish to, prove that they have been injured as a result of someone else's negligence. Establishing the cause of disablement for the remaining 90 per cent of disabled children is virtually impossible. For the relatively small number of children who successfully pursue claims for compensation through the courts, awards are made on the same basis as for adults. As with social security benefits the presumed object of compensation is the child herself or himself, though it could be argued that compensation is also owed to the family.

Given this balance of congenital and acquired disabilities, the

Pearson Commission made the decision that, unlike disabled adults, children with severe disabilities should be treated as a homogeneous group, no distinction being made between them according to the cause of their disablement.

In considering ante-natal injury, we found that the cause of such injury could rarely be established with certainty. There are some 90,000 severely handicapped children whose condition is due to congenital disability, but only those whose condition is caused by injury before or at birth are within our terms of reference. These children cannot be distinguished from those whose condition is caused by genetic abnormality or disease, and it is simply not within our terms of reference to devise a separate scheme of compensation for the children who are within our terms of reference.[62]

Hence, in the case of disabled children the Commission went beyond its terms of reference to consider both existing and desirable provision for all disabled children whatever the cause of the condition.[63] Since the legal system, as we have seen, provides for only a tiny minority of cases this meant primarily looking at the social welfare system. What was provided and how far it appeared, to the Commission, to be adequate is considered below.

State provision for disabled children

As with disabled adults, state support for disabled children takes a variety of forms, the central divisions being between statutory and voluntary sources and between financial help and services in kind. Here we consider only statutory sources – the cash benefits provided by the social security system, and services in kind provided through health, education and personal social services, with the Family Fund in a somewhat ambiguous place between the two. Considerable support is provided through the voluntary sector but this is too heterogeneous to consider here.

Social security

The cash benefits provided through the social security system do not address themselves particularly to the situation of disabled children and their families. The only cash benefits children are eligible for – attendance and mobility allowances – are a comparatively recent development in the system of cash help for disabled people, being independent of a national insurance contribution record and aiming, not to replace earnings, but to help with costs arising from disablement. When they were introduced, children crept in under the adult umbrella. There seemed no good reason to exclude them, but there is no evidence that when these first cash benefits ever paid to disabled children were introduced, this was the result of hard thought about the needs of disabled children as a group. The somewhat arbitrary age and disability criteria adopted for both benefits support this view.[64]

Until the introduction of these benefits, social security provision for 'civilian' disabled people had been geared to providing a basic income in lieu of earnings. However the social security system does not compensate loss of earnings by adults caring for a disabled child unless family income falls below the basic minimum embodied in the supplementary benefit scale rates and in means-tested benefits for low earners. Disabled children themselves do not lose earnings and, like the legal system, the social security system focuses on the disabled individual rather than on the carer or the family unit as a whole. So there is no mechanism at present for explicitly compensating families with a disabled child for loss of parental earnings. There is also resistance to compensating married women for caring for dependents; this conflicts with assumptions, deeply embedded in the social security system, about the financial dependence of married women on their husbands and about the division of labour within the family. Married men are seen as responsible for providing the family's income; their wives as occasionally supplementing that income but primarily responsible for the nurturing of children and the care of dependents. Hence married women living with their husbands are excluded from the scope of the only benefit – the invalid care allowance (ICA) – which compensates people who have given up or are unable to start work because of caring for disabled relatives. (Women with disabled children who are divorced or widowed *do* qualify for ICA.)[65]

Services for disabled children

Services for disabled children have been described in detail elsewhere and it would not be appropriate to summarize that account here.[66] They have a long history and strong connections with voluntary and philanthropic activity, though at the present time both statutory and voluntary agencies are involved in their delivery. The range of services that exists is very wide. However the level of support provided to the majority of families with disabled children seems to be much less than the theoretically wide range of services available would suggest.

The fragmentation of services for disabled children prior to the establishment of the new integrated local authority social services departments in 1970 makes it difficult to judge the quality of provision for their families. However a number of research studies in the 1970s indicated that provision was poor, as did the Younghusband Report in 1970.[67] Though Sir Keith Joseph originally asserted during the Thalidomide debates that the special needs of disabled children were being adequately dealt with by the statutory authorities, this view had to be revised in the course of the parliamentary debates. Both in those debates and in the 1974 House of Commons Paper it was acknowledged that existing services were not adequate.[68] Research into needs and services undertaken by the Family Fund research team between 1974 and 1976 confirmed this view, as did research from other institutions.[69] Hence the Pearson Commission, having looked at all the evidence on the quality of existing services for families with disabled children, and particularly at the work done by the Family Fund research team, concluded that as sources of help or compensation they were not significant:

> Local authority provision under the relevant legislation covers a wide range of services. In practice the amount of help given varies considerably among the different authorities. It includes services provided by social workers, residential care, special fostering and boarding-out arrangements, adaptations to houses, aids and telephones.
>
> No reliable estimate can be given of the value of local authority services currently provided to severely handicapped children, but it is probably less than £1 million a year. We have the impression that local authorities, in distributing their limited resources, tend not to give high priority to provision for severely handicapped children.[70]

The Family Fund

The Family Fund, the organization set up in 1973 in the wake of the Thalidomide affair and administered by the Joseph Rowntree Memorial Trust, had an initial budget of £3 million to complement existing provision from statutory and voluntary services. The initial £3 million was followed in 1974 by a further £3 million. The amount of help disbursed by the Fund since then has settled down to around £2.5 million a year. The Family Fund has been the subject of a detailed evaluation by Bradshaw who concluded that as an organization it had advantages over other methods of giving help to families with disabled children, including the fact that its particular focus on the needs of families, and the disabled child within the family, was appreciated by the families themselves. Nevertheless, Bradshaw argued, the Family Fund's flexible and discretionary method of help could only be justified 'as an adjunct to a system of clearly delineated rights based on principles of equity'. There were three reasons for reaching this conclusion. First, the Fund was 'inadequate to meet the gap in provision that it was set up to fill.' Second, only a third to a half of eligible families had applied for help. Third, the whole nature of the Family Fund's discretionary, philanthropic dispensing of help on the basis of individual decisions by social workers was inequitable.[71]

The Family Fund does not, therefore, fill the gaps in existing social security and service provision for disablement in children. The shortfall was acknowledged by the Pearson Commission: 'Even when account is taken of all the existing forms of support, a gap remains.'[72]

To help close that gap Pearson recommended improvements both in services and in the cash help available: a new general expenses benefit of £4 a week (at 1978 prices) and the extension of the mobility allowance to children under five and those whose mobility problems did not stem from purely physical causes.[73]

There has been no increase in the real level of cash support for disabled children and their families since the Pearson Commission reported in 1978. This can be attributed partly to deterioration in the economy since that time and partly to the practical difficulties of introducing an expenses allowance only for children with disabilities. It may also be a consequence of the fact that the rationale for compensating families with disabled children has not been explicitly argued in any major policy document. As we have already observed, the Pearson Commission did not argue the case for the increased support it recommended. The following chapter therefore examines the claim disabled children and their families have on the community at large and their rights to compensation from the state.

2 Disabled children – rights to compensation?

Whether and why the state should provide support to people 'in need' is a topic which currently absorbs both policy-makers and academics in the fields of social policy and political theory.[1] This preoccupation with the normative basis of state welfare reflects the disappearance of the consensus that existed in post-war Britain, and until fairly recently, as to the necessity and value of a collectively-financed 'welfare state'. In the absence of a shared ideology of welfare the pursuit of logically-defensible principles is inevitable – and invaluable.

In the following pages, then, the claim that disabled children and their families have on the state and on society at large is examined in some detail.[2]

The central issues involved are succinctly summarized by Plant:

> Broadly speaking, there are two views on the question of the moral basis of welfare provision. One is that welfare is a matter of charity, generosity, humanity; of giving but not of strict obligation. The corollary of this view is that the recipients have no moral rights to what they receive because no individual person can have a right to another person's charity. The other view is that welfare is a matter of strict obligation for those who hold resources and that those who are in need have strict moral claims on those better-off in society.[3]

On which side of this divide does the help provided to disabled children lie? Is severe disablement in a child a purely private misfortune and help provided purely out of compassion? Or is there any sense in which disabled children have 'strict moral claims' on society?

The nature of society's obligations towards disabled children and their families is examined here for two reasons. First, to provide a conceptual framework within which the appropriate policy response to any financial losses experienced by families with disabled children can be discussed. Second, because the issues involved are relevant to the question of responsibility for the care of dependent people generally. At a time when 'community care' policies increasingly attempt to place responsibility for the care of highly dependent people on their families, it is useful to re-examine the extent of collective responsibility for dependency and how far compensation is owed to those who discharge obligations which belong in part to society as a whole.

In the following pages, then, a number of different accounts of the basis on which help is, or should be, given to disabled children and their families is examined and the problems raised by some of these accounts discussed.

The argument from compassion

Perhaps the first response evoked by our question is that help is given to disabled children and their families because their situation touches us. Awareness of their needs creates a desire to help. Behind this response lie views of children as vulnerable and precious and parenthood as the desire of most people. Disablement in a surviving child is unexpected and the more painful because of its relative infrequency. So, it is argued, the majority of people want both disabled children and their parents to have whatever will help to ease their distress and restore their lives to something approaching normality. On this view, help is a pure gift – an expression of compassion. Such views are often linked to ideas about the value of 'community' and how welfare based on altruism rather than rights and obligations enhances the lives of the people who give and receive help and promotes feelings of community.[4]

There are two serious problems in attempting to base the provision of support to families with disabled children on compassion or altruism. First, it is difficult to envisage the support of dependent people being adequately provided in complex industrial societies on the basis of compassionate response. In even a small town it is difficult to ascertain the needs of individuals beyond one's own network of acquaintances or immediate geographical locality. It is certainly impossible to tap the feelings of individuals and organize the efficient delivery of support without using the machinery of the state or some other organization. Hence sympathy alone is an unreliable source of help, particularly when help is needed on a prolonged or intense level. Neither private nor organized charitable activity can guarantee the kind of help on which people in need can confidently base their lives. Altruism is 'perhaps too insecure a basis on which to base the life-chances of the disadvantaged.'[5]

The second problem is that if help is provided from compassion the people for whom compassion is felt have no rights to help and those who feel (or do not feel) compassion no obligation to help or to see that help is provided. Such a view carries with it the possibility, not only of inadequate provision, but of stigma for the recipient:

> If it is accepted that welfare is to be seen as a form of charity and institutionalized generosity, then it would seem that the recipients of welfare, understood on this basis, might well feel that their receipt of benefits could be stigmatizing. . . . If those in need have no right to the resources of others, other than an appeal to their generosity or humanity, then it is difficult for them to avoid being put in a subordinate status of dependency on others.[6]

Clearly, then, there are problems in proferring compassion alone as the basis of the help provided to disabled children and their families.

The argument from social justice

It is tempting to ground the case for supporting families with disabled children in arguments about justice. However such arguments inevitably lead to the necessity of defining the concept of justice that is being used. Are we, for example, talking about justice as a single, unitary, concept or about a group of principles which together constitute a working notion of justice? If the latter, which are the salient principles? Are we, for example, talking of justice as the protection of rights and liberties; the reward of deserts; the meeting of needs; fairness; or as treating individuals with equal respect? Titmuss identifies four maxims which, for him, constitute 'the historic principles of distributive justice':

1 To each according to his need
2 To each according to his worth.
3 To each according to his merit.
4 To each according to his work.[7]

These he regards as defensible, though sometimes competing,

principles which together add up to social justice. Other writers base their notions of justice on particular principles. Walker, for example, equates justice with equality and, drawing on Durkheim, Tawney and Marshall, elaborates a theory of citizenship according to which justice for disabled people can be identified as access to citizenship rights on an equal footing with non-disabled people.[8]

The problem with such views lies in their use of what have been described as 'contestable' concepts.[9] That is, concepts such as equality embody values rather than empirically ascertainable or logically testable facts. Hence it is impossible to validate accounts such as Walker's because the meanings he gives to terms such as 'justice' or 'equality' can be contested by people with different views.

Such problems would not arise if agreement could be reached on the nature of justice as a single concept, rather than a body of principles each of which is contestable. However the attempt to formulate an objective account of social justice as a unitary concept has not, to date, succeeded.[10] Indeed the search for such an absolute conception seems misguided; ideas of justice are inevitably bound up with particular ways of looking at society, and reflect contemporary values.[11]

It seems unlikely, then, that the case for helping disabled children and their families can convincingly be based on the concept of social justice.

Need

It is often asserted that the meeting of needs is the principal function of social welfare systems. On this view collective responsibility to provide help for disabled children and their families exists because disablement creates special needs. However the existence of a need is not sufficient to act as an unequivocal claim on public resources. The concept of need, as Bradshaw and others have pointed out, is both complex and contestable.[12] It has even been argued that 'need' is a meaningless concept and should be replaced, in policy discussion, by the concepts of wants and preferences.[13] At the very least, the ends for which particular items are necessary have to be specified before it can be decided to allocate resources to satisfying them.[14] The problem is that many types and levels of need exist and some of them are indistinguishable from wants. Whether they are accepted as making a legitimate claim on collective resources must often be dependent on subjective points of view. 'The classification of needs is going to depend, crucially, upon ends, goals and purposes the justification of which is an ineradicably moral enterprise, and one that may be morally contestable.'[15]

Since meeting one individual's needs can involve diminishing the welfare or invading the property rights of others it is clearly desirable to reach agreement on the needs, if any, that constitute a legitimate claim on other individuals or on the community at large.

There is some agreement that basic human needs can be identified, that the obligation to meet these is a strict duty and that the legitimacy of governments is bound up with their fulfilling this strict obligation to meet the basic needs of all citizens. However basic needs are usually defined only as what is needed for survival and autonomy.[16] When we start to discuss what autonomy means in a particular society the debate again becomes a matter of value judgments.

The arguments examined so far have not provided a convincing account of the basis on which help should be provided to disabled children and their families. In the remainder of this chapter we explore the extent to which collective responsibility for helping such families can be established and grounded in a theory of human rights.

Rights to welfare?

Whether there are rights to welfare or to a certain level of material well-being has been the subject of considerable debate in recent years among political theorists and academic lawyers in particular.[17] It is argued below that such rights do exist and provide a firm basis for the claims of families with disabled children both for support by the state and to compensation in the sense identified by Titmuss.[18] First, however, we discuss why rights claims are stronger than claims based on compassion, justice and need – and why they are resisted.

The particular importance of rights claims is that they are capable of validation – by reference to law or custom or by logical argument. Claims based on rights are not weakened, therefore, by subjectivity. Jones identifies three reasons for the popularity of rights language in the field of social welfare. First, they are claims with a special force: to claim a right is to say that one is entitled to something without further argument. Second, the existence of rights justifies the state in raising revenue, which may be unpopular. Third, receiving welfare as a matter of right is more dignified than receiving it as charity.[19]

As noted earlier, the idea that there is a human right to welfare, in the same sense that there is a right to life, for example, or to a fair trial, is strongly resisted. It is argued, for example, that social and economic rights belong to a completely different logical category from the traditional human rights and that to treat them as the same weakens the status of these traditional rights. It is also objected that meeting the social and economic rights of poorer individuals involves unacceptable infringements of the property rights of the better-off. A less common objection, associated with Titmuss in particular, is that treating welfare as a right, rather than as a gift, harms rather than enhances human and community relations.[20]

In spite of these objections it is possible to argue a convincing case for the existence of human rights to welfare. However this is an absolute right only to a minimum level of provision – whatever is necessary for survival and autonomy. Beyond that, though moral rights can exist to a higher level of provision, these are weaker and can legitimately be weighed against competing claims on resources. This second stratum of 'rights' has been variously characterized: as ideal rights, conditional rights, aspirations and so on. Describing them as rights indicates that they have a claim, though not an over-riding claim, on community resources and governments a duty to meet them as soon as possible.[21]

What is important for our purposes in this debate is the acknowledgment of the existence of moral rights to welfare, not confined to the positive rights enshrined in existing statutes. Though individual claims may have to be assessed in the light of other claims, claims to welfare as a right cannot be reduced to mere rhetoric.

Jones identifies three types of moral right to welfare: rights held as human beings and citizens; insurance or contractual rights; and rights to compensation, held against the state.[22] In the case of disabled children and their families all three can be argued to exist. Disabled children's moral rights to welfare are discussed further below. Before this, however, it is necessary to introduce a clarification which lies behind much of the ensuing discussion.

This consists of making explicit that, though disabled children and their families have so far been treated as though their rights and interests were identical, this is not necessarily so. Disabled children and their parents have their separate rights as human beings and these may conflict. Securing the rights of very dependent children can involve a heavy burden of care for parents. This may in turn affect parents' ability to obtain things which are taken for granted in this society, some of which are regarded as human rights. This might include, for example, rest, leisure, paid employment, participation in the social and political life of the community and an end, in time, to the obligations of parenthood.

Conflicts of rights are not novel. It might simply be argued that if the parental rights that are jeopardized are not fundamental human rights (such as the right to life) there is no strict obligation on society to protect them. However if society does have moral obligations towards disabled children, which are partly discharged by parents, it would seem that it has a duty to investigate the costs experienced by parents in discharging these obligations and, as far as possible, to compensate these. This depends, of course, on disabled children's having rights to welfare and society's having the reciprocal duty of honouring these. Do such rights exist? And on what grounds?

Disabled children – human rights to welfare

The rights of disabled children to support from the state originate in their right to life. Once it is established that the state has an obligation to secure their right to life it would seem to follow that the obligation of providing care also falls partly to the state.

The right of children with very severe disabilities to life is acknowledged and protected by the state by both direct and indirect interventions. Indirect intervention takes the form of allocating resources to the development of highly specialized medical facilities. Without these many severely disabled children would die; their existence makes survival possible, but at a very high level of dependency. Direct intervention takes two forms. First, where parents refuse consent for routine procedures which doctors wish to perform and without which children would die, the state may assume parental powers and authorize the procedure. For example, Alexandra, a child born in 1981 with Down's syndrome, had an intestinal blockage which was simple to remedy but fatal unless operated on. Her parents refused consent for the operation. However at the request of the doctors involved the local authority intervened. The child was made a ward of court and her care and control given to the local authority. Second, people who take steps actively to prevent even very severely disabled infants from surviving may be prosecuted for murder or manslaughter. Again in 1981 a paediatrician was tried for allowing severely impaired new-born children to die, with the consent of their parents.

The debate prompted by these cases indicated that a great deal of uncertainty existed, both about the desirability of prolonging the lives of severely impaired infants and about the *locus* of responsibility for decision-making. Alexandra's right to life was upheld by the High Court; the paediatrician who had allowed severely impaired infants to die was acquitted. Both decisions appeared to command general assent.[23] What was clear, in spite of this ambivalence, was that society continued to assert an interest in decisions about the survival of such infants. There was no consensus that doctors should allow profoundly impaired infants to die. Nor was the right to decide whether their lives should be prolonged by medical intervention assigned to parents. Parents' wishes were clearly subordinated both to the prevailing social ethic and to the judgment of doctors. Since maintaining life subsequently involves not only medical and other professional resources but also heavy burdens of care, it seems obvious that both parents and child have a right to support with these burdens for the remainder of the child's life.

The problem with this argument is that it does not lead to a *general* responsibility on the part of the state towards all disabled children, but only towards those whom medical technology has saved or where there has been direct intervention to preserve life. Investing resources in medical techniques which will preserve life suggests *some* responsibility for the subsequent quality of life; the difficulty lies in the fact that the general right to life does not appear to impose strict obligations on states or societies to develop any particular set of medical techniques. Nor can it be argued that the decision to develop one type of medical intervention implies a positive affirmation of the superior rights of one set of individuals to life. This decision appears, therefore, not to imply a strict responsibility for the subsequent maintenance of life including the domestic burdens of care. (The more dramatic cases of individuals who would have died had not the state intervened does seem to imply responsibilities of this sort; however such cases are numerically few and the responsibilities usually acknowledged.) If we are looking for an account of collective responsibility towards all disabled children it is probably preferable to base this, not on the commitment implied in the commitment of resources in medicine but instead on general human rights to survival and autonomy. This implies that disabled children – and by implication all severely disabled people – have the same right as non-disabled people to look to the state as guarantor of their survival and, implicitly, of whatever is necessary for autonomy. That the costs of this may be greater for people who are severely disabled is irrelevant.

On this view it can be argued that the duty of maintaining life, including the subsequent burdens of care this implies, falls ultimately to society at large rather than to families or friends. It may be desirable that families carry some of these burdens However they do so partly on behalf of society and have a right, therefore, to support or to compensation for the losses they suffer as a result.

It is possible, however, to postulate a quite different version of society's responsibility. On this view the care of dependents is primarily a kinship obligation and the responsibility of the state only to ensure that arrangements exist for the care of very dependent people. These arrangements will normally take the form of care by families, the state having a duty to step in only when families are unable to cope.

The scope of the issues raised by these different stances is potentially enormous. They reflect very different and probably irreconcilable views of the origins, functions and value of state welfare – topics far beyond the scope of this book. They also reflect different views of family and kinship obligations for the care of dependents. Since this dispute is of central importance in eliciting what is owed to families caring for disabled children it is necessary to reflect, briefly, on the extent of family responsibility for the care of dependents.

Dependency, the family and the state

State–family relations and the division of responsibilities for the care of dependents are perennial concerns of politicians and social scientists. Both are concerned with the extent to which the caring functions formerly thought to be performed by families have been transferred to the state. This preoccupation has assumed increasingly urgent political dimensions in post-war Britain because of two parallel and opposing developments: an increase in the total volume of dependency and a simultaneous drop in both public and, it is argued, private provision for it.

The rise in dependency stems from an increase in the numbers of elderly people relative to the population of working age and an increase in the number of people of all ages surviving major illnesses and severe congenital impairments but remaining highly dependent. The reduced capacity of families to provide care is argued to have three causes: the virtual disappearance of the 'domestic spinster'; greater geographical mobility; and changes in the behaviour and aspirations of women in relation to paid employment, together with the compression of child-rearing into a much shorter period. The reduced capacity for public care has two sources. First, attitudes towards care in residential institutions have altered. They have come, increasingly, to be viewed as offering an inferior life to that 'in the community'. Second, a succession of economic crises has been accompanied by a reduction in the resources available for residential care without an accompanying increase in the amount available for care in the community.

The evidence that the net effect of these changes has been to move responsibility to any extent from the family to the state is far from clear. On the contrary, a number of studies suggest that families provide a growing amount of care. Moroney, for example, found 'no evidence that the family as such is giving up its caring function'.[24] Particularly in the wake of community care policies, Moroney found families to be providing the bulk of care to their dependent members. Though a consensus existed that responsibility for dependent people ought to be shared, in reality support to families was minimal and concentrated at the point where the family's caring capacity broke down and institutional care was sought.

In practice, then, it seems that families are bearing heavier burdens of dependency rather than transferring these burdens to state agencies. Is this reasonable? Or is there a case that in devolving its own responsibility onto families the state is acting unfairly?

The responsibilities and rights of parents with disabled children are more easily discussed in the context of child-raising generally than of disability or dependency: different things are expected of families in relation to children, adults and elderly relatives.

The relationship between parents, children and the state can be represented as a dichotomy with, on one side, children as the exclusive responsibility and 'property' of their parents and, on the other, the 'Brave New World' nightmare vision of children as the entire responsibility of the state – nurtured outside the family as a future work-force and acquiescent citizenry.

In reality, of course, the relationship is better represented as a continuum along which provision in different societies can be ranged. Kamerman and Kahn, in a study of family policy in fourteen countries, characterize three main types of family policy: explicit and comprehensive; explicit but with no overall goals; and implicit and reluctant. The United Kingdom is placed in the last category, though as Land and Parker point out the absence of 'an integrated set of social policies explicitly termed family policies'[25] should not conceal the fact that Britain has an implicit policy towards families, underpinned by its own ideology and with its own purposes.

Briefly, in Britain families are expected to bring up children with a minimum of help (or 'interference') from the state. The day-to-day job of bringing up children falls mainly to parents, who are expected to bear the costs of child-raising in return for the benefits this brings. The family is regarded as a private domain and as an institution which, though performing vitally important social functions, is also fragile and must be protected from anything that might undermine it. Two of its most important functions are socializing future citizens and providing care for dependent members. The traditional division of labour within the nuclear family – men earning and women providing care – is seen as the most efficient (or 'best') way of carrying out these functions. Social policies in Britain tend to support this implicit model. What actually goes on in families stays largely invisible. Non-intervention is justified by the family's vulnerability in the face of bureaucratic meddling.

This non-interventionist policy has consequences for the welfare of all families with dependent children. However some of the heaviest costs of a privatizing ethos which places responsibility for children principally with their families are borne by families with severely disabled children. Their parenting task is more demanding than that of parents with normal children and their need for support correspondingly greater. However in the absence of a well-developed ethos of shared responsibility for all children, adequate support for families with disabled children is less likely to develop.[26]

It is not difficult to demonstrate that the notion of the family as a private domain is untenable. The state intervenes extensively in family life. Families are extensively regulated to secure various ends for the state and society at large.[27] It is difficult, therefore, to sustain the view of the family as a private sphere where parents have full rights over, and therefore full obligations for their children's lives. The state's interventions, which are neither disinterested nor politically neutral, create reciprocal obligations towards *all* families with children. In the case of severely disabled children its active role in protecting their rights to life makes it difficult to argue convincingly that the obligation for providing care can legitimately be devolved onto families without support or compensation.

This view is strengthened by the fact that care by families means, almost exclusively, care by women, and that a conflict of rights exists between carers and cared-for in which the state has duties towards both. That women's rights are at risk within families was recognized in the nineteenth century by minds as diverse as those of Engels and Mill.[28] Today there is much more general assent to the view that the rights of women should be protected. Equal Opportunities and Sex Discrimination legislation impose a duty on governments to ensure that those rights are not systematically violated.

It might be argued that the roles of wife or mother carry obligations which transcend women's own rights as citizens or human beings or the positive rights to equal opportunities which they have under the law. However, this position is difficult to sustain once a collective duty to preserve the rights of disabled children to life is recognized. Allowing the care of dependents to fall, uncompensated, on women threatens both their human rights to (equal) autonomy and the positive rights secured in legislation. It would seem, therefore, that the state has a particular obligation to ensure that the rights of women caring for dependents are protected, at least by providing compensation for their loss of earnings or realistic payment for the caring job they do.[29]

Parents of disabled children themselves point to the lack of compensation at present for the burdens they carry and which they might legitimately transfer to the state by placing their children in residential institutions. Many parents in the present study argued that, since families caring for severely disabled children at home are saving the community the considerable costs of institutional care, some of these savings should be channelled back to families: in payment for the caring job they do; in compensation for the stress and opportunity costs experienced by different family members; and to help prevent family breakdown.

The difficulty with this argument is that, though placing a child in residential care is theoretically an option, a number of pressures prevent its being an automatic right or one that many parents would in any case wish to exercise. The circumstances in which families are allowed to abrogate their duties towards dependents are relatively few and controlled both formally, through rules and tests, and informally through stigma:

> Many policies are built on an implicit assumption that the extended family is the dominant structure and by definition this family is viewed as generally self-sufficient in meeting the needs of its members. The healthy family is one that does not seek support from extra-family institutions and for a family to do so is an admission that their support network is inadequate. When it breaks down the social welfare system intervenes on a residual basis. The State, for example, can take over certain functions or even completely substitute for the family when it is seen as incapable. Usually some sense of stigma is attached.[30]

The stigma will be stronger in relation to children than to elderly relatives. Putting children in care is seen as much less legitimate in present-day British society than having a parent in an old people's home. So the notion that any family with a disabled child may simply choose between the options of assigning the child to the care of the state or looking after her at home, with an implicit right under the second option to compensation from the savings this creates, is not entirely realistic. It does, however, have some validity, which is strengthened by an examination of the reasons why the option of assigning the child to the state's care is not freely available.

First, the great majority of parents with disabled children simply prefer to keep their children at home with them. They love their children. They are also influenced by the value attached to parental responsibility for children in Britain and share the prevailing view of the illegitimacy of abandoning their responsibilities. This view is, however, reinforced by a number of factors. Some of these relate very directly to government policies, making parents' decision to look after their children at home not wholly a private decision but one which the state implicitly encourages them to make.

One strong influence encouraging parents to keep their children at home is the narrow range and generally poor quality of residential care available. Parents' own perceptions of the poverty of residential care available are reinforced by two professional streams of knowledge. The first, which originates in the work of Bowlby,[31] stresses the importance for the child of maintaining close contact with a limited number of adults. The second, drawing on the work of Goffman[32] and others, stresses the diminishing effects of institutions on the individual. These ideas provide the basis of the views professional workers transmit to parents of institutions as bad places for children. The principle that it is in the best interests of the child to be at home is deeply embedded both in professional theory and in government policy, where it is used, for example, as one of the justifications for community care policies. At present it is increasingly difficult to find permanent residential places or respite care for even the most severely disabled children. To the extent that government policy actively deters parents from seeking residential care for reasons that are partly to do with cost, families who bear the costs of providing care at home have a moral right to compensation.

It would seem then that a strong case can be made for the existence of a human right to welfare on the part of disabled children themselves. Moreover by virtue of discharging privately what is partly a collective responsibility the parents of disabled children also have rights to support or compensation. This is not the only ground on which disabled children and their families have claims on society. As noted above, a moral right to welfare also exists in two other circumstances: when certain risks are collectively insured against and when responsibility for a disadvantage belongs to society as a whole. Both can be argued to arise in the case of severe disablement in children.

Insurance rights and the redistribution of burdens

A central value of modern welfare states, and one which the state has a duty to express, is that burdens should not be distributed too unequally. Risks are pooled and collective provision made so that excessively heavy burdens are not privately borne by small minorities.

Severe disablement in a child is a contingency which is rare, not easy to prevent or predict, and creates considerable burdens for families. As such it is clearly the kind of contingency that welfare states are established to provide for. In this respect, therefore, families with severely disabled children have a right to expect the burdens created by disablement to be shared. As citizens and taxpayers they would be correct in viewing the child's disablement as a contingency collectively insured against, and both cash benefits and services as forms of support to which they have rights.[33]

Compensation rights against the state

It was noted earlier that[34] compensation rights can be invoked against the state when society generally can be held responsible for an individual's disadvantage. This argument originates in the concept of social costs developed by the economist Pigou in the 1920s[35] and subsequently applied, by Titmuss in particular, to British social policy:

> The notion of social costs recognises that all the costs of producing a good or service are not borne by the producer, and that all the costs involved in the enjoyment of consumers' goods or services are not borne by the consumer in question.[36]

Their unequal incidence creates a case for equalizing the adverse effects of production – that is, compensating those on whom these adverse effects fall.

Disablement in children provides a clear example of the unequal distribution of social costs and the case for compensation can be argued at a number of levels.

First, some disabilities can be traced directly to advances in medical technology. Titmuss cites the classic case of blindness induced in some new-born babies by the administration of high oxygen concentrate:

Towards the end of the 1940s, as a result of scientific and technical advances (or changes) in medicine and allied fields, some maternity hospitals began to administer high oxygen concentrations to certain newly-born babies. In 1954 the *Lancet* drew attention to the fact that this 'scientific advance', while benefitting some babies, had caused 'an alarming increase' in the number of babies who, after some months, were found to be otherwise healthy but totally blind.[37]

Similar examples readily spring to mind – vaccine damage and Thalidomide damage, for example – and a case is easily made for compensation being due to people disabled as a result of technological advances which have benefited the community at large. The technologies which have, as a side effect, injured some children have enabled others to live normal lives who would otherwise have died. Compensation for the accidental victims of technological progress seems inherently reasonable.

Second, though it is impossible at present to establish exactly what the 'causal agents' are, it is probable that some congenital disabilities arise as a by-product of advanced industrial technology. Pollution from industrial plants, both air- and water-borne, car exhausts, pesticides, contact with toxic materials by pregnant women, and even the general stress induced by working in noisy factories, may all affect the health of unborn children. The difficulty of identifying causes precludes, as we have seen, the pursuit of compensation through the courts and supports the case for compensation by the community at large. It, after all, benefits from economic growth and advanced technology.

Third, there is evidence that much congenital disablement can be attributed to the failure of the state to prevent it. That increased expenditure on ante-natal screening and services, improved special care facilities and better-organized maternity services would reduce the incidence of congenital disablement could be argued to place some responsibility for compensation on the state which has a duty to prevent disablement when ways of doing this are known to exist.

Conclusion

It seems, then, that disabled children and their families can establish rights to support or compensation from society at large on the grounds discussed above. This is not to say that compassion, justice and the meeting of needs are of no relevance to their situation, but that claims based on rights have certain advantages – notably that they are capable of independent validation. It will often be preferable to use the language of rights since claims based on rights are more difficult to set aside when there are competing claims on resources.

It may seem unnecessary or invidious to assert that disabled children and their families have rights to payment or compensation. It might be feared, for example, that emphasis on the rights of carers will deny that there is a place for the unselfish exercise of care and compassion within families and in the community at large. This anxiety seems unfounded. The meeting of rights leaves ample room for the exercise of generosity and may in some circumstances be a precondition for it. The possibility of loving relationships within families seems more at risk from heavy physical burdens and the necessity for constant self-sacrifice than from the provision of adequate help, provided as of right before the point of breakdown is reached. The securing of rights need not encroach on the sphere of human relationships that is characterized by generosity and unselfishness, either within families or between families and the wider community. As Kleinig points out, both are necessary for 'adequate moral relations'.[38]

The arguments presented in this chapter suggest that disabled children and their families have strong moral rights to adequate support and compensation and the state a strict obligation to honour these. What has not been discussed is the particular form or level such compensation should take. Decisions have to be made about the balance of cash and support services, for example, and about whether the state should provide cash compensation for pain and suffering, or only for earnings-loss and extra costs. Such decisions can only be made in the light of the resources available, and knowledge of the effects severe disablement in a child typically has on family life.

The study reported here was concerned to establish empirically the extent to which families were affected financially by severe disablement in a child – in the language of the tort system, the extent of any pecuniary losses. The following chapter discusses the methodological problems of doing so.

3 Measuring the costs of disablement

Measuring the extent to which a child's disablement affects families financially is not a simple task. Disablement can affect the economic functioning of an individual and of the family to which she belongs in a great many ways. Its effects can also spill over beyond the immediate household – to extended family members living elsewhere, to the local neighbourhood and to the community at large, through the provision of statutory and voluntary services and through the loss of output of disabled people themselves and of those whose employment is affected by the need to care for them. The discussion that follows concentrates on the effects experienced by the disabled individual and the immediate family. It encompasses both children and adults with disabilities. Clearly, however, there will be differences in the effect according to the age of the disabled person and his or her relation to the labour market.

The legal system of compensation provides a useful summary of the financial consequences that can follow from disablement, since its purpose is to make good those consequences. This system recognizes that disablement can have effects that are financial and some which are not straightforwardly financial, but involve pain or loss of faculty. Into the first category fall earnings loss – for the person who is disabled and for relatives or friends needed for care. Extra expenses – both obvious and hidden – can arise. The burden of caring can also make demands on the time of relatives or friends, creating what economists call 'opportunity costs'. What may be understated in this account are the diffuse spillover effects of disablement, flowing from the time and energy consumed in caring: the need to pay for routine jobs that would previously have been undertaken by family members, for example. More expensive shopping and compensatory spending on non-disabled siblings can also arise because of pressure on parental time. Even effects not directly associated with loss of money, such as loss of faculties like sight or walking ability can, as the tort system recognizes, carry financial implications. To lead as full a life as possible can cost more.

All these, then, are possible and intuitively reasonable consequences of disablement. All are recognized and have been compensated in the civil courts for well over a hundred years. Demonstrating empirically that they do arise, and quantifying their level poses difficult problems however – both in the choice of research method and in the interpretation of findings.

Earnings loss, for example, may seem fairly easy to establish since comparative earnings figures are usually available. Even so, it presents problems. It is not always possible, for example, to separate the effects of disablement from other reasons for low earnings. Moreover effects on earnings may not be confined to the disabled person but cause complicated alterations in the behaviour of other family members. The disabled person may be at home, and hence free another family member for paid work. Alternatively she may need so much care that someone has to give up paid work or reduce the hours they work. In the case of disabled children, reduced earnings by mothers may be offset by increased earnings by fathers.

Decisions about work and leisure and the allocation of time between the two are complicated in any household. Theoretical analysis of these decisions indicates that they are strongly influenced by the earnings that can be commanded by different household members, the value of their time to the household and the value of their leisure time.[1] Disablement will further complicate these decisions. Where someone is disabled, complicated arrangements may be made between household members to allow both caring and the earning of the necessary income.[2] Decisions may have to take into account the stress and isolation of the carer, and may well be influenced by the availability of cash benefits paid on account of disablement. Hence in estimating earnings loss it is the earnings and behaviour of the family or household as a whole that have to be considered – in the case of disabled children the earnings of both parents. For crude earnings figures this does not present insurmountable problems. Establishing and quantifying the opportunity costs of the household – the time spent in caring and what its value would have been to the household or the individuals concerned – is much more intractable. How is one to measure the decrease in the efficiency with which the household is run because of the time and stress involved in caring for a disabled child or making it possible for a disabled adult to go out to work? Or, conversely, how can one measure the increase in the efficiency of household organization which some women with disabled children may achieve as a result of not going out to work? People adjust in complex ways to disablement in a family member, working out their own strategies to minimize its effects on both income and psychological well-being. These adjustments, together with hidden costs, may mean that earnings figures alone are not an accurate indicator of the extent to which living standards have been affected.

Quantifying effects on expenditure poses greater problems. Above all, the tastes and preferences of individuals and families vary so much that it is difficult to draw inferences about relative living standards from expenditure figures. Even where the problem is not complicated by disablement, the use of expenditure data to measure living standards or the cost of bringing up children is both problematic and controversial.[3] The introduction of disablement as an additional factor produces yet more complications. The notion of 'extra' expenditure depends on ideas of normal expenditure which may be too simplistic, given the wide variation that average expenditure figures frequently conceal. What is normal expenditure for one person will be 'extra' for another; one person's necessity will be another's expendable luxury. Moreover spending depends on having money to spend and being physically able to spend it. There will be disabled people who stay cold because they cannot afford heating, and people who spend very little on entertainment because they are unable to go out alone or cannot find someone to look after the disabled person. In neither of these cases will the amount spent be a reflection of needs or preferences. And the same amount of money may purchase very different quantities of a commodity for disabled and non-disabled people. Five pounds spent on taxis or buses buys very different mileages or numbers of outings. Five pounds spent on ordinary groceries buys more than it would of special diabetic food. Here again expenditure cannot be taken as a measure of utility. Nor is additional spending always strictly necessary. It may be absolutely necessary; it may, on the other hand, be incurred in improving the quality of the disabled person's life or minimizing the effect of disablement. And, as with earnings, families will adjust their expenditure patterns to the special demands created by disablement in ways that are difficult both to track down and to interpret. There may be a switch from spending on luxuries for the whole household. Alternatively, the disabled person's standard of living may be maintained at the expense of other members of the family. Some families will cope by developing extremely efficient housekeeping strategies which others may be unable to afford – as in bulk buying – or simply lack talent for. The distribution of money within the family may alter, so that wives have access to more of the family's income than they would otherwise have done. The extended family, too, may provide more help in cash or in kind than would normally have been the case.

Apart from the difficulties created by these different coping strategies, problems arise in deciding the time period to which expenditure should be related and in dealing with the fact that it can be very frequent or intermittent, planned for or unpredictable and urgent. A final difficulty is in evaluating expenditure on goods which, while they cannot really be afforded and might not be wanted, do increase families' standards of living: cars, washing machines and other 'luxury' consumer durables.

Measuring the financial impact of disablement in a family member is, then, fraught with problems. These problems have been dwelt on at this stage to demonstrate that since the financial consequences of disablement are so complex and so diffuse it is difficult to encompass all of them in any one study. The consequences can evolve and alter over long periods of time, the adjustments and coping strategies of families may vary enormously. The condition itself will be only one of the factors shaping their response.

Hence the financial effect of disablement can be studied in a number of different ways and from a variety of perspectives – ranging from the detailed personal accounts of individuals to statistical analysis of data on large populations. There is no perfect methodology. There are, as we shall see, gains and losses from each. Methods which are ideal in theory – for example longitudinal comparative studies based on expenditure records maintained over long time periods – are unworkable in practice. The choice of method will depend, crucially, on the purposes of the research and on the resources available. These, together, will determine the study's approach.

A very broad distinction can be made, however, between two approaches to measuring the financial effects of disablement. They can be studied from the subjective perceptions of the people immediately affected or they can be studied by comparing the incomes and expenditure patterns of households with and without disabled members. Neither method is without weaknesses. The distinction allows us, however, to see how, in the case of the present study, the approaches used in previous studies were inappropriate – both ideally and because they did not meet the requirements of our policy customers in the DHSS.

Previous studies of the financial consequences of disability

Looking broadly at the literature on the financial consequences of disablement it is possible to make three generalizations:

1. Effects on income have been investigated much more often than effects on expenditure and have used a mainly comparative approach; studies of expenditure effects have invariably been subjective.
2. There has been much more detailed study of the effects of disablement in adults on family incomes than of disablement in children.
3. Very few studies have looked simultaneously at income and at expenditure effects.

Information on the financial impact of disablement in adults has come both from large-scale statistical studies of poverty and income distribution and from smaller studies looking specifically at disabled people. The picture that emerges from both is remarkable in its consistency over time. Among large-scale studies the pioneering work was that of Abel-Smith and Townsend who in their analysis of Family Expenditure Survey (FES) data for 1953–4 and 1960 revealed that disablement was strongly associated with low income.[4] This finding was confirmed in the 1969 OPCS survey[5] and again by Townsend's major survey of poverty in the United Kingdom, the fieldwork for which was carried out in 1968–9.[6] Most recently it has again been confirmed by an analysis of data from the 1975 General Household Survey (GHS), commissioned by the Royal Commission on the Distribution of Income and Wealth.[7]

Among studies specifically of disabled people, Sainsbury's early work in charting the effects of disablement on the incomes, and to some extent the expenditure patterns of a sample of people with disabilities has been confirmed both by the 1969 OPCS survey and by a number of smaller studies, many commissioned by pressure groups such as DIG and the Disability Alliance.[8] The clear picture conveyed by all these studies is that being or becoming disabled has a marked effect on income. Lower earnings are not offset to any extent by social security transfers. In spite of new benefits, disabled people remain disproportionately represented among the poor, while a high proportion of the disabled have very low incomes. Even when they are not technically in poverty, disabled people are likely to find their incomes lower as a result of disablement. This is not only a British phenomenon. Large-scale longitudinal work carried out at the University of Michigan indicates that in the United States too, disablement is a major cause of poverty.[9] Little is known of the extent to which reduced earnings by a disabled family member are made good by altered work patterns in other family members, though data from the 'misfortunes' survey carried out by the socio-legal studies unit at Wolfson College, Oxford, suggest that this does not happen to any extent.[10]

As has already been noted, attempts to gauge the effects of disablement on (adults') spending patterns have been universally subjective in approach. People with different types and degrees of disability have simply been asked whether they think disablement has affected how they spend their money and why this happens. In some cases they have also been asked to estimate their 'extra' spending on a given range of items or to discuss needs which cannot be met because of lack of money. This approach has been used in a large number of studies, ranging from general studies of the effects of disablement such as those of Sainsbury and Blaxter[11] and studies sponsored by pressure groups,[12] to Harris's large, representative 1969 survey.[13] The picture that has emerged from all these studies is of fairly large proportions of disabled people claiming that their disablement necessitates extra spending or creates a need for extra spending which cannot always be afforded. A third of respondents to the 1969 survey, for example, claimed to have at least one extra expense because of their disablement; one in fifty claimed to have three or more such 'extra costs'. This subjective approach has provided much useful information on the ways in which disablement can alter expenditure patterns and on families' coping strategies. While it has the merit of being a fairly simple technique to use, it is not unproblematic and its disadvantages are discussed below.

Two characteristics stand out in research on the financial effects of disablement in children. First, the lack of comparative data extends to incomes as well as expenditure patterns. The labour-force participation of women with and without disabled children has been compared in a number of studies.[14] However the effect of women's altered employment patterns on families' incomes has been derived only from parents' subjective estimates. The true level of differences in mothers' and fathers' earnings and the extent to which these are mitigated by social security benefits has remained unexplored, with the exception of an analysis of data from the General Household Survey (GHS) by Piachaud et al.[15] In this analysis the participation rates, hours of work and earnings of families with and without disabled children in the 1974 GHS were compared and found not to differ significantly in most respects. The number of disabled children was very small, however, and the results are therefore suspect. Effects on expenditure have, to date, been explored solely through the perceptions of parents with disabled children themselves.[16]

Second, information on the financial implications of disablement in children has emerged from general studies of the impact of disablement rather than from 'purpose-built' studies. Burton's study of children with cystic fibrosis, for example, Hewett's study of cerebral palsied children, and Woodburn's study of children with spina bifida were all general studies which included questions on the financial impact of the condition. Among studies of general populations of disabled children (as opposed to studies of children with particular conditions) the work of Butler and his colleagues at Bristol[17] and of the Family Fund research team[18] again took the form of general surveys including a few questions on earnings effects and the need for special expenditure. Very few studies have addressed themselves specifically to the financial consequences of disablement; those that have have focused on particular conditions or particular problems – Bodkin et al.'s work on the costs of childhood cancer, for example, or Kew's work on the costs associated with hospital treatment.[19]

In general these studies suggest that the work and earnings of the majority of women and of a significant number of men with a disabled child are adversely affected; that the great majority of families experience at least one 'extra cost' and that most experience more than one. Seventy-eight per cent of the families in one Family Fund research team study, for example, said that the earnings of at least one parent had been affected. This study, which was based on a postal survey of 361 applicants to the Family

Fund, found no respondents who said they had no extra costs because of the child's disability; 73 per cent said they had more than one.[20]

Research of this type is of limited use in planning policy and establishing whether there is a case for improvements in cash benefits – whether for children or adults with disabilities. It leaves unspecified the level of any extra spending and, in the case of children, the magnitude of any earnings loss by parents. Nor does it convey anything about the combined effect of earnings loss and extra expense. Two studies, one of children and one of adults, have carried the subjective approach a stage further than the studies described so far and, in doing so, have filled in some of these gaps.

In a follow-up survey of applicants to the Family Fund 303 families were asked, in 1975, whether the child's condition had affected mothers' or fathers' earnings or had caused extra expenditure. Where it had parents were asked to estimate their weekly earnings loss and their extra spending on a range of items.

Of the families in this sample 48 per cent said that their earnings were less because of the child's special needs, the average weekly loss of earnings being estimated at £20.40. Ninety per cent claimed to be spending extra on at least one of the items for which precise figures were requested. The average extra amount spent each week on these items was estimated at £2.10. (All at 1975 prices.)[21] This study shares the drawbacks of subjective assessments of earnings loss and extra costs discussed below. However it was a first step towards establishing the magnitude of effects on earnings and expenditure patterns.

Hyman's study of the extra costs of disabled living for 56 adult wheelchair users developed this approach further in an attempt to obtain a comprehensive picture of the costs imposed by disablement.[22] Her study not only included detailed estimates of earnings losses and all extra expenses, but also measured the opportunity costs of close relatives and friends and the costs borne by the community at large in the form of services and cash benefits. The particular strengths of Hyman's study were its comprehensiveness and the fact that the comparatively small sample and the use of only two very experienced research workers meant that her estimates of costs and income losses were much more rigorously worked out than in previous studies. Moreover the case-study approach allowed Hyman to assess the total financial effect of disablement on individual families. This study provided ample evidence of effects on earnings and of additional spending necessitated by disability. However the small numbers, the study's limited geographical coverage,[23] and the narrow range of disabilities covered meant that Hyman's findings had limited applicability.

Even Hyman's approach is not free from the shortcomings inherent in subjective accounts of the financial impact of disablement. They assume a degree of consciousness about the way money is spent which is probably unreasonable. They rely, too, on an unlikely degree of knowledge of what respondents' income and expenditure would have been or of what 'normal' income or spending is for people not disabled. They are made even more unreliable by the variety of individual preferences and priorities for spending money. Such calculations have, therefore, all the weaknesses of hypothetical estimates based on imperfect knowledge.

Additional difficulties arise from questioning parents directly about the effect of disablement in a child on their finances. Some parents may be reluctant to claim any financial effect, because they are unwilling to blame the child for the family's financial difficulties, or want to stress the child's normality rather than point to differences. Others, alternatively, may claim that the child's condition affects them financially because they feel this is the answer the researcher wants or because they are under stress in other ways. That is, to a degree greater than with less sensitive topics, answers to subjective questioning about the financial effect of disablement may be influenced by emotional factors which are impossible to account for in analysing replies. There will also be cases where, though families probably do experience both costs and earnings losses, money itself is regarded by parents as unimportant in the context of caring for children who are suffering or dying. Some parents are under such stress that they are almost completely unaware of what they are spending. They are unlikely to be capable of accurately assessing how much more their food or heating costs are than those of similar families without a disabled child.

It might reasonably be argued that many of these problems arise with all surveys using interviews and particularly where information on expenditure is elicited by direct questioning. However the estimation of earnings loss and extra expenditure caused by disablement relies to a much greater extent than is usual on calculations based on hypothetical and untestable notions of what might have been. They are therefore subject to stronger reservations.

The comparative approach

Given these reservations about the reliability of subjective estimates, measuring the financial impact of disablement by comparing incomes and expenditure patterns in families with and without disabled children has clear advantages. The particular value of comparative data is that, being concerned with what people actually earn or spend, rather than what they think they do, they provide a clearer picture of differences between families with and without disabled children. If families are not different in other respects, differences in incomes and expenditure patterns can be attributed to disablement.

While using comparative data resolves some of the problems of using subjective impressions, it is not without disadvantages of its own.

First, comparative data has its own problems of accuracy and reliability. The information obtained is still dependent on recall and will often depend on the maintenance of detailed expenditure records – a taxing task for busy people. Forgetfulness or deliberate falsification may lead to the over- or under-recording of certain types of expenditure: special expenditure for the disabled person, for example, or 'stigmatizing' expenditure such as alcohol or tobacco. Finally, the survey itself may change respondents' behaviour so that what is recorded is not typical.[24]

Second, as we have already observed, the financial consequences of disablement are neither simple nor uniform – either between families or over time. Hence comparative data from one point in time has limitations which may seriously diminish its validity. Choosing to study actual behaviour and to concentrate on current income and expenditure must inevitably result in a loss of valuable information that could be elicited by more subjective questioning about disability and families' response to it. Cross-sectional surveys cannot provide information on events that have happened in the past, for example. So they cannot tell us about expenses that occur spasmodically or about episodes of financial stress associated with disablement and which families without a disabled child would not experience – hospitalization, the cost of moving house, paying for structural alterations to a house, buying special equipment and so on. Perhaps only a longitudinal study would pick up and make sense of such episodes thoroughly. Subjective questioning can at least uncover their existence and how common they are.

Another important aspect lost by the comparative approach is the process by which disablement affects earnings and spending patterns and, even more important, the processes by which people adapt to it. *How* does severe mental handicap in a child come to affect expenditure on food or clothing? And why in some families and not in others? How do families react to such extra costs? Men may seek higher-paid employment, which may in turn cause extra stresses for the woman who stays at home. This and other coping strategies may have 'costs' and consequences for other family members and, arguably, for social policy. They are, however, impossible to isolate from the bare statistics yielded by comparative survey material. In some ways comparative data on incomes and current spending may conceal as much as it reveals.

A related problem, touched on already, concerns the interpretation of these bare statistics, and of expenditure figures in particular. Suppose, for example, that a sample of families with a disabled child records expenditure on transport no higher than that of a similar group of families without a disabled child. This might suggest that disablement did not affect transport expenditure. Behind that, however, lie a number of special factors that affect being able to spend on transport. Some people may record little or no expenditure because they cannot afford it; some might be unable to benefit from going out, or be unable to manage alone and so 'save' money – which means they can find the extra money needed for another item; some will spend the same amount as the comparison group but get much less utility for it because they have to travel by taxi, which is more expensive than public transport. So the expenditure recorded cannot be taken as an accurate measure of consumption or as an indicator of need. Disablement may impose such constraints on spending that comparisons of this sort are not appropriate. In addition different types and degrees of disablement affect spending in different ways, which makes it difficult to compare incomes and expenditure patterns for the sample as a whole. It *is* possible to look at individual commodities for different sub-groups of the disabled sample. However, this leaves the very

60 *Measuring the costs of disablement*

difficult problem of building up a picture of the expenditure patterns of the disabled as a group, or the total financial impact of disablement on an individual family. The latter certainly calls for a much more subjective, case-study approach as does any attempt to understand the meanings families give to their situation, their coping strategies or the help, if any, they feel is appropriate for them. These limitations mean that the financial impact of disablement is inadequately described by comparative data on its own. Ideally a mix of comparative and subjective approaches is required. In the case of the study reported here, as the following chapter shows, the constraints of the policy-making process also dictated that such a mix of methods be used.

4 The study – design and methods

The subjective approach of previous studies greatly limited the usefulness of their findings for practical policy-making purposes. While indicating that disablement in a child reduced most families' incomes and created extra costs, earlier research had not provided information reliable and detailed enough for policy development. Most importantly it had not demonstrated conclusively that the financial stresses reported by parents of disabled children were greater than those experienced by other families with children. Before cash benefits for disabled children could be improved policy-makers in the DHSS wanted to be sure of the case for doing so. This meant demonstrating that the incomes and expenditure patterns of families with disabled children differed substantially from those of families with normal children. A new study, which would contain a comparative element, was therefore commissioned.

In theory, comparative data could have been obtained by mounting a purpose-built survey comparing the incomes and expenditure patterns of a sample of families with disabled children and those of a control. However practical considerations of cost and timing ruled this out. It was decided instead to obtain information on the incomes and expenditure patterns of a control group of families with children from an existing data source – the Family Expenditure Survey (FES). To provide comparable information for families with a severely disabled child this survey would be replicated for a sample drawn from applicants to the Family Fund.

Neither the Family Fund nor the FES was without disadvantages. The Family Fund was established in 1973 to give help to families with a severely disabled child. Applicants were a self-selecting group who might not be representative of all families with severely disabled children.[1] The Family Fund register was, however, the largest and most comprehensive available sampling frame for severely disabled children at the time of the study, containing information on over 40,000 applicants.

The FES is a continuous government survey providing information annually on the incomes and expenditure patterns of a representative sample of households in Britain. FES, which is described in detail in the survey handbook,[2] has two main elements: an interview, in which details of income and certain recurring expenditures are collected, and a diary record of all household expenditure in the 14 days after the interview. As a source of information on the financial impact of disablement FES shares the limitations of comparative data discussed in the previous chapter. It has additional limitations of its own. For example, it does not gather information on important topics such as disablement or the services families receive. It also records expenditure in ways that make it difficult to isolate expenditure on the disabled child from that on other members of the family.[3] For these reasons FES on its own would not yield reliable information on the financial impact of a child's disablement. Comparative data from FES would need to be supplemented by subjective information from parents.

The new study's design therefore had three discrete elements.

A comparison of incomes and expenditure patterns

A slightly modified version of the FES was administered, between January and July 1978, to a sample of families with severely disabled children, drawn from Family Fund records. Data on these households' incomes and expenditure patterns were compared with similar data from a group of families with children who had taken part in the routine FES during the first six months of 1978.

Additional information

The entire sample of families with disabled children was asked an additional set of questions. These questions had three main purposes:

> To provide information not collected in FES but of central importance to this study – on the child's condition, for example, and families' receipt of benefits and services.
> To investigate costs which arose infrequently and for which FES

data was unreliable – consumer durables, for example, and adaptations to housing.
To guide interpretation of the statistical material from the comparative part of the study.

Case studies

Important ways in which the child's condition had affected families financially would inevitably be missed in a large-scale survey whose emphasis was on the current situation. Nor could structured interviews conducted by professional interviewers capture the complexity of families' individual circumstances or the overall effect of the child's condition on their finances. For these reasons some 10 per cent of the families with disabled children were followed up and interviewed in depth.

The families with disabled children

Sample size and coverage for the comparative study

Both cost and the practical difficulties of replicating the complicated fieldwork operations of the FES limited the sample of disabled children to around 500. The FES control was unlikely to be larger than 700. These are small samples for the task of measuring the financial impact of disablement in a child. Expenditure in particular is so variable that differences found in the two samples' expenditures might be due to sampling error rather than the child's condition. It was therefore necessary to find ways of reducing sampling error. This was done in two ways. First, the coverage of both samples was restricted, both geographically and in terms of family composition. Only two-parent families, living in England, with a maximum of three dependent children and no adult non-dependents were selected for interview. Second, in order to reduce variation caused by factors other than the child's condition the samples were matched on important variables. Ideally, the sample of disabled children would have been drawn so that it matched the FES sample on five variables, all of which influence expenditure: the regional distribution and timing of interviews, social class and the number and ages of children. For a number of reasons, not least the impossibility of knowing the characteristics of the 1978 FES families in advance, it was possible

64 *The study – design and methods*

to attempt matching only for region, class and the timing of interviews when the sample was being drawn. Further matching was done at the analysis stage. (Sampling is discussed in more detail in Appendix 1.)

Fieldwork

Families who appeared from Family Fund records to meet the criteria for inclusion in the study were approached by letter, via the Family Fund. This letter explained the study's purpose and the criteria for familes to be interviewed and asked them to participate if they still met these criteria. A reply slip was enclosed to return if families no longer fitted the criteria or were unwilling to participate.

Fieldwork for the main study, including the coding of questionnaires, was carried out by Social and Community Planning Research Ltd. Their brief was to replicate the procedures used in FES. In this they had advice and guidance from the Office of Population Censuses and Surveys (OPCS) which has responsbility for FES up to and including the coding of questionnaires.

Response

It was imperative that the number of interviews successfully completed with parents of disabled children should not fall far below 500. This meant devising a method of drawing the sample which allowed non-respondents to be replaced by similar families and monitoring response throughout the six months fieldwork period. (These procedures are described more fully in Appendix 1.)

Table 4.1 Response of families with disabled children

	No. of families
Approached	842
Not traced	84
Not eligible	145
Unwilling to participate	120
Not interviewed – other reasons	5
Successfully interviewed	488*

*Eight of these were excluded from the final sample because of missing information or unsatisfactorily completed expenditure diaries. The final total of successfully completed interviews was therefore 480.

The study – design and methods 65

In all, 842 families with disabled children were approached, to produce a final total of 480 completely successful interviews. This does not mean that the response rate for the study was poor. As Table 4.1 shows, the commonest reasons for 'non-response' were that families' circumstances made them ineligible for interview or that they could not be traced. The true response rate, calculated from the number of eligible families asked to participate, was around 78 per cent.

The FES control group

A sub-sample of the 1978 FES tape containing information on a group of families with dependent children was obtained from the Department of Employment. Like the sample of disabled children, the FES sub-sample included only single tax-unit families living in England, interviewed in the first half of 1978 and comprising two parents and up to three dependent children at the time of the interview. This sub-sample numbered 712 families. Fifteen families were subsequently excluded: seven because they were found not to meet the criteria for the study and eight because evidence of benefit receipt and attendance at special schools suggested that a child in the family might be severely disabled. This left a total of 697 families.

As in other research projects information on the incomes of families where the breadwinner's main source of income was from self-employment was found to be unreliable. Data on these families was therefore excluded from the analysis, leaving a total of 438 families with a disabled child and 638 control families.

The depth interviews

We had intended to draw a quota of families to be interviewed in depth randomly from each month's successfully completed interviews in the comparative part of the study. However, this resulted in children with only the commonest disabling conditions being selected. We therefore selected a number of children with less common conditions from each month's completed interviews, drawing the remainder of the quota randomly. In all 56 families were approached, of whom 48 agreed to be re-interviewed.

The families in the study

We turn now to the families who finally took part in the study, looking first of all at similarities and differences between the families with disabled children and those in the FES control and going on to discuss briefly the characteristics of the disabled children themselves.

We had attempted to match the samples on three variables: their regional distribution, the timing of interviews and social class. Since neither the characteristics of respondents to the 1978 FES[4] nor of the families with disabled children who would agree to participate could be known in advance there was no guarantee that this attempt would succeed. In the event, there was no difference in the regional distribution of the two samples. However the timing of the interviews differed slightly, fewer of the disabled children's parents than of the control group being interviewed in January and correspondingly more in June. This meant that there might be slight discrepancies in the two groups' incomes (because of wage increases and changes in tax and benefit levels in the budget) and expenditures (because of seasonal variations in prices and inflation). It would have been possible to make adjustments to the data to correct most of these discrepancies. However scrutiny of the changes in prices, earnings and tax benefit levels that actually took place in the first six months of 1978 indicated that these were slight. It was unnecessary therefore to adjust the data to take account of these differences.[5]

The attempt to match the samples' social class composition at the sampling stage was less successful. This was largely because the Family Fund classifies occupations using the Registrar-General's six-point classification[6] while the FES uses an eight-point classification based on, but not identical to this. Matching could therefore only be attempted on a broad non-manual/manual distinction. In the event even this was not successful, mainly because of differences in the way the two systems classified certain occupations as non-manual or manual. In consequence the occupation group structure of the two samples was different, the families with disabled children having significantly more men in manual occupations. (See Table 4.2.)

This difference in occupation structure was mainly of significance in the comparison of men's earnings. In comparing men's earnings care was therefore taken both to estimate the effect of

Table 4.2 Occupation group structure*

Occupation group	Families with a disabled child		FES control	
	No.	%	No.	%
Professional and technical workers	31	7	100	15
Administrative and managerial workers	41	9	95	14
Teachers	8	2	26	4
Clerical workers, e.g. clerks, commercial travellers, agents	34	7	31	5
Shop assistants	3	1	4	1
Manual workers: skilled	220	47	274	40
semi-skilled	108	23	130	19
unskilled	24	5	22	3
Total	469	100	682	100

*FES occupation groups.

differences in occupation structure and to take account of it. In general comparisons were made only between men in the same occupation groups and between men in manual and non-manual occupations, rather than for the samples as a whole. (Differences in occupation group structure are discussed in more detail in Appendix 1.)

As noted above, the samples would ideally have been matched on two aspects of household composition which have an influence on expenditure: the number of children and their ages. In practice this was impossible – partly because the characteristics of the families who would take part in the 1978 FES could not be known in advance but also because for families applying to the Family Fund this information is collected at the time of application. It would therefore have been out of date by the time the sample was drawn.

There were differences between the samples in both respects. The families with disabled children contained fewer one-child and more three-child families. There were also significantly fewer young children in this sample, largely because Family Fund policy tends to exclude families where the disabled child is under two. (The sample of disabled children in fact contained no children under two.) As far as possible these differences in family composition were taken into account in analysing both income and expenditure data. Differences in the number of children presented no problem. It was relatively simple to look at families with one, two and three children separately. The age distribution of the children was more problematic. One solution would have been to exclude all families with a child under two from both samples. This would have involved an unacceptably high loss of cases, however, since there were non-disabled children under two in many of the two- and three-child families with disabled children. It was decided not to exclude these families permanently from the study but to attempt to ensure, in analysing the data, that groups of children of similar ages were compared.

The disabled children

In setting up the Family Fund the government restricted its scope to children who were severely disabled. Criteria for establishing what constituted disablement severe enough to make families eligible for help were established by the Fund itself in consultation with a panel of consultant paediatricians. The result was a set of guidelines rather than hard and fast rules. For example spina bifida was judged to be severe if it involved paralysis of lower limbs and incontinence of urine or faeces; mentally handicapped children were usually eligible only if their IQ was less than 50; severe hearing impairment had to involve 'severe impairment or complete loss of hearing with marked communication problems'. A number of moderate disabilities could add up to disablement that was severe overall; handicapping factors such as attendance needs, especially in the night, could also be taken into account. Each child's individual circumstances were to be considered on the basis of the information supplied by parents to a visiting social worker from the Fund. Where there was doubt as to eligibility medical corroboration would be sought – initially from physicians who knew the child and ultimately from the panel of paediatricians advising the Fund.[7]

The children in this study were all severely disabled according to Family Fund criteria, while more than 95 per cent of them also met the criteria for the attendance allowance. Like any sample drawn from the Family Fund this group contains children suffering from a wide range of conditions (see Appendix 1). It also includes both mentally and physically disabled children. Half of the children were judged to be severely mentally handicapped. Some of them suffered from a single impairment such as deafness or blindness;

the vast majority were multiply disabled.[8] The average number of disabilities they suffered was five; 10 per cent of them had only one or two disabilities and 12 per cent eight or more. Not surprisingly, most of these children were very dependent on others in matters of self-care and in moving around. Over 80 per cent required help with washing, dressing, feeding, toileting and moving around indoors.

Statistics such as these give little idea of the individual children concerned. We therefore conclude this chapter by briefly describing the disabling conditions suffered by five of the children whose parents were interviewed in depth.[9]

Andrew was fifteen at the time of the study and very severely disabled. He was completely paralysed, spastic, doubly incontinent, had no speech and suffered from chronic bronchitis. He also had an inoperable hiatus hernia which caused frequent vomiting. Andrew was not mentally handicapped and fully understood what was said to him but was able to communicate only by grunts or whines.

Martin was six and had congenital Thalidomide-like deformities. He had twisted rudimentary feet at about mid-thigh level but they were at such an angle that he could never hope to walk with them. He used them instead as levers and moved rapidly around indoors with the help of his bottom. Outdoors he used heavy artificial legs or a wheelchair. One arm ended in a stump; the other, his best limb, was missing some fingers. Martin was very dependent on his parents in matters of self-care and for getting around.

Joyce was twelve and suffered from cystic fibrosis (CF) – an enzyme deficiency which causes excessive quantities of mucus to be produced. In CF the pancreas progressively becomes shrunken and replaced by fibrous tissue so that the digestion of fats is affected. Obstruction of the mucus glands in the lungs leads to infections, bronchopneumonia and lung abscesses.

The prognosis for children with CF is very poor. Most die in their teens and many before. The common picture of life for a CF child is of chronic digestive problems and frequent chest infections, each of which inevitably increases lung damage and shortens life expectancy. Joyce was not diagnosed as having CF till she was five and already very poorly, with some lung damage. She suffered from frequent chest infections, stomach pains and diarrhoea. She was extremely thin, pale and very frail and was unable to attend school at all.

Jason was eight, suffered from spina bifida and hydrocephalus and was slightly mentally handicapped. He was paralysed below the waist but could walk a few steps with the help of a walking frame when wearing full-length calipers. He was doubly incontinent and also suffered regular severe attacks of bronchitis which caused breathing difficulties and vomiting bouts. Most of these problems were exacerbated by his being greatly overweight.

Anna was thirteen and severely mentally handicapped. She was hyperactive, aggressive and generally very disturbed in her behaviour: unpredictable, stubborn and very difficult to manage. She appeared to have no conception of right and wrong and would, for example, torment animals, smash furniture and break windows. Anna was tall and very heavy which increased the difficulties of coping with her. She was partially incontinent and frequently experienced *grand mal* epileptic fits.

These, then, were some of the children whose effects on their families' finances were the subject of this study. The chapters that follow do not explicitly describe the ways in which bringing up children like these is more taxing than the normal job of bringing up children. Other studies have done this.[10] What is assumed here is that severe disablement in a child is usually associated with prolonged dependency; with increased contact with hospitals and other agencies; with intermittent illness and other crises, and hence with increased demands on parents' time and energy. In the following chapter we examine the extent to which this heavier parenting task affected families' incomes.

5 Incomes

In this chapter the effect of disablement in a child on income is examined by comparing the incomes of this sample of families with disabled children with those of the families in the FES control. This comparative material is illustrated by information obtained in interviews with the parents of disabled children themselves. We begin by comparing the two groups' gross incomes and the source of their incomes.[1]

Gross incomes

As Table 5.1 shows, the gross incomes of the families with disabled children were £6.40 a week less, on average, than those of the control families. The distribution of income in the two groups was also very different, fewer of the families with disabled children having very low or very high incomes.

Table 5.1 Gross incomes

	Families with a disabled child £ per week	Control group £ per week
Mean	110.3	116.7
Lower quartile	89.8	85.9
Median	105.9	109.0
Upper quartile	127.6	135.7
No. of families	438	640

It was known that the proportions of manual and non-manual workers in the two groups was not the same. This meant that it would be necessary to investigate whether these differences were real or simply a reflection of the samples' different occupational structures. This is done below (see pp. 90–5 and 99–106). For the moment we look at the sources from which families' incomes were obtained.

Sources of income

Two things emerged from looking at the sources of families' incomes (see Table 5.2). First, *all* the components of their original incomes were smaller for the disabled group than for the families in the control. Second, the largest differences between the two groups occurred in earnings and in the level of social security payments. Compared with these differences, those in unearned income were fairly trivial. Since, in addition, relatively few of the families in either sample had substantial unearned income, our analysis concentrated exclusively on earnings and social security payments.

Here, as Table 5.2 shows, differences between the two groups were substantial. The earnings of the families with disabled children were lower than those of the FES control group, and formed a smaller proportion of total family income; social security payments were larger for the disabled group and formed a much larger proportion of total income.

Table 5.2 Sources of income

	Families with a disabled child		Control group	
	Mean £ per week	% of income	Mean £ per week	% of income
Earnings	84.1	76	103.0	88
- women's earnings	6.5	6	14.6	13
- men's earnings	77.6	70	88.5	76
Social security payments	21.0	19	5.4	5
- for disability	14.0	13		
- other	7.0	6	5.4	5
Imputed income	4.6	4	6.5	6
Income from other sources	0.7	1	1.7	2
No. of families	438		640	

Earnings

For the families with a disabled child parental earnings, at an average of £84.10 a week, made up 76 per cent of their gross weekly incomes. For the control parental earnings, at £103 a week, were £18.90 more and constituted 88 per cent of income. This difference was not unexpected. Less predictable was whether the overall difference in parental earnings would be caused primarily by differences in the employment patterns of mothers or in those of both parents.

As Table 5.2 shows, the lower earnings of the families with a disabled child were caused by differences in both men's and women's earnings. Among the families with a disabled child women's earnings made up 6 per cent of total family income; the figure for women in the control was 13 per cent. The earnings of the men with a disabled child formed 70 per cent of family income, as against the 76 per cent share contributed by the earnings of the men in the control. In money terms the earnings of the women with a disabled child were £8.10 a week lower, on average, than those of women in the control; those of the men with a disabled child £10.90 a week lower than the earnings of their FES counterparts.

Looking at earnings figures for the sample as a whole in this way leaves many questions unanswered. How general is earnings loss among men and women with a disabled child? Are the observed earnings differences the result of different participation rates or of differences in the number of hours worked? Or are they the result of differences in hourly rates of pay, indicating that it is the type of job held that is different? Who is bearing the brunt of any differences in earnings – those who are poorly paid, or those who are by some standards more able to withstand some earnings loss? Not least, what is it about disablement in a child that causes earnings loss and why do some families lose earnings while others are unaffected?

With these questions in mind we turn now to examine the employment patterns of men and women separately. Women's employment patterns are examined first, since by virtue of their traditional caring role there is a *prima facie* case that they will bear the brunt of any earnings loss within the family.

The work and earnings of women with disabled children

The most fundamental change in the structure of the labour market in Britain, in the post-war period, has been in the employment patterns of married women with children. There is a wealth of statistical evidence to demonstrate that it is now the norm for women to be in paid employment for a large part of their 'working' lives – giving up full-time employment typically with the birth of their first child and returning, often initially to part-time work, as their children become more independent or suitable care arrangements are found.[2]

Alongside this statistical evidence of married women's increasing participation rates is a substantial body of evidence that their earnings now play a key role in maintaining the economic welfare of their families. Women's earnings are not, that is, a fringe benefit increasing family income to the point where some luxuries and a generally higher standard of living become possible. For the majority of families with working wives, the wives' wages are necessary if the family is to have a reasonable standard of living. For around a million families with children it is the earnings of wives which bring them above supplementary benefit level – the officially defined poverty line.[3]

The research that has been done on married women's employment patterns suggests that the decision to seek work outside the home is influenced by the age and number of children in the family, by the husband's earnings, the pay women themselves can command and also by a number of less easily quantifiable factors – the availability of jobs with suitable hours, suitable childcare arrangements, whether there is a local tradition of women working, support from husband and family, and so on.[4] A constantly recurring theme in much of the research on this topic is that, for many working mothers, the task of combining the roles of parent and wage-earner is very difficult. The analysis of women's employment in the present study has to be set in that context. Women with disabled children presumably encounter the same imperatives to seek paid work as other women with children do, and face all the problems encountered by women with children in trying to enter the labour market. They have, additionally, to deal with the problems created by the child's disablement.

It is intuitively credible, then, that the extra stresses and complexities brought to family life by disablement in a child will deter many women from going out to work – even though, paradoxically, isolation and financial strain may increase their desire to do so. Previous studies have invariably found the majority of mothers saying that the child's disablement affected their working lives;[5] comparative data on the economic activity of women with children in the general population tends to support this view.[6]

The present study allowed us both to examine the basic questions of whether and how the work patterns of women with disabled children differed from those of similar women with healthy children, and to go beyond this to questions not tackled in previous studies. In particular the financial effect of different participation rates and how this varied at different stages of the family life-cycle were examined.

Labour-force participation, hours and earnings

The participation rates, hours and earnings of the women in the two samples were very different (see Table 5.3). The women with a disabled child were much less likely to go out to work: 33 per cent of them, as against 59 per cent of women in the control, were in paid employment at the time of this study. When women with a disabled child did go out to work they worked fewer hours and earned correspondingly less than employed women in the control. As Table 5.3 shows, the women with a disabled child worked on average four hours less and earned £7.10 a week less than women in the control.

Table 5.3 Characteristics of women's paid employment[7]

	All women	Age of youngest child		
		0–4	5–10	11–16
Participation rate (%):				
Women with a disabled child	33	25	38	44
Control group	59	42	72	87
Mean weekly hours:				
Women with a disabled child	19	16	20	20
Control group	23	18	22	28
Mean weekly earnings (£):				
Women with a disabled child	22.1	18.2	24.1	21.7
Control group	29.2	23.9	26.9	38.0

Whether women with children go out to work and the number of hours they work are both known to be strongly influenced by the age of their youngest child.[8] When there is a pre-school child in the family relatively few women go out to work. As children grow up mothers' labour-force participation and hours of paid work increase. This suggested that the overall differences in employment patterns observed above might be obscuring the pattern of differences between them at different stages of the family life-cycle. It seemed likely that the employment patterns of the women in the two samples would be most similar when children were young and would increasingly diverge as they grew older.

This expectation was confirmed. As Table 5.3 shows, whatever the age of their youngest child, fewer women with a disabled child were in paid employment, they worked fewer hours and earned less than similar women in the control. However differences in employment patterns increased markedly with the age of the youngest child, reaching their maximum when the youngest child was eleven or over. At this stage 44 per cent of the women with a disabled child, as against 87 per cent of the women in the FES control, were in paid employment. Those who were in paid employment worked on average eight hours fewer than the women in the control and earned an average of £16.30 a week less.

These differences in weekly earnings largely reflect the shorter working week of the women with a disabled child. They also reflect the more subtle influence of shorter hours and less continuous labour-force participation on hourly rates of pay and lifetime earnings potential. The average hourly earnings of women employees with a disabled child were 14 pence less than those of those in the control. Moreover, whereas the hourly rates of the latter increased as children grew older, those of the women with a disabled child actually fell slightly. By the time all the children in the family were eleven or over the difference in women's hourly earnings had increased to 27 pence.

These earnings figures, then, show the financial penalty paid by women with a disabled child for remaining much longer than the women in the control group in part-time work. There is no doubt that when women with disabled children in the present study were able to go out to work at all, only part-time work allowed most of them to care as they wanted for the disabled child and the rest of the family. They typically sought work as school-dinner attendants, barmaids or cleaners. However, such jobs are low-paid and part-time working implies a wide range of disadvantages apart from low pay. A number of studies have shown how it is typically associated with poorer working conditions, less security of employment and exclusion from benefits such as sick pay, paid holidays and superannuation.[9] Most women employees with children experience these disadvantages when their children are young but increase their hours of work and move back into jobs with training and career structures as their children grow up. When all the children in the family were eleven or over 43 per cent of the women in the FES control as against 15 per cent of the women with a disabled child were in full-time work. Clearly, women with a disabled child are less free to increase their hours of work outside the home, with a consequent effect on lifetime earnings and employment conditions as well as on current earnings.

In the following section we look more closely at how disablement in a child affects a woman's ability to earn – drawing extensively on the views of the women in the study.

Very few of the women who were interviewed in depth about the effect of their child's disablement on their employment outside the home said that this had been wholly unaffected – only 7 out of 48. Four of these women had other young children and recognized that this would have constrained them anyway. Two were working part-time and had no desire to work full-time. The seventh was a nurse who had always managed to find a nursing job that would fit in and who had very supportive relations living nearby – though even she acknowledged that, ideally, she would have liked to be a theatre sister and could not fit that in with her daughter's needs.

The commonest reason given by mothers in these interviews for their work being affected were the number of things that had to be done for the child, and the difficulty of finding people willing or able to look after her after school, in illness or in school holidays. Apart from physical dependency, the aspects of disablement mentioned most often as preventing mothers from working were the child's difficulty in communicating basic needs to unfamiliar people, the difficulties of management created by hyperactive behaviour, and the child's own need for intensive stimulation, teaching or exercises of various sorts. The fact that time off was frequently, and sometimes unpredictably, needed because of hospital appointments or illness made mothers reluctant to commit themselves to employment, while the sheer fatigue of caring for some children, especially those needing frequent attention at night, made such a commitment unthinkable. (Not only could some of these mothers not contemplate going out to work; they could not manage the disabled child and other household responsibilities without regular help from their husbands.)

Typically, mothers gave a cluster of reasons for being unable to go out to work, as the following cases demonstrate. The mother of a fifteen-year-old quadriplegic and very dependent spastic boy, with two other children over ten, explained how her son's condition meant that she was unable to work, though she had at one time been a well-paid clerical worker:

> 'First of all, in the morning Andrew's got to be got up and dressed and fed and toileted, and you know he's got to be *held* on the toilet – you can't leave him. It's a couple of hours, really. And you can't do anything else while you're feeding him. If you turn round, it's spat out. It's a couple of hours getting him ready for school. And then when he comes home at half-past three your time is devoted to him. Someone has to be there. And when he goes to bed you're constantly turning him. He has to be turned so many times before he goes to sleep. And he can be sick three times a night. . . .'

This boy was often ill and was sometimes sent home, quite unpredictably, from school. Not surprisingly, his mother felt that she needed the time when he was at school to organize things for herself and the rest of the family.

The mother of a nine-year-old child with advanced muscular dystrophy and confined to a wheelchair was similarly prevented by the demanding job of caring for him from contemplating work outside the home. He had to be carried around indoors, especially to the toilet, needed someone to pick up the things he frequently dropped, had to be fed and also talked to and stimulated. His mother was up with him, turning and toileting him six or seven times in the night and had to be up at six-thirty to start getting him ready for school. After school he could never be left on his own in the house in case he hurt himself.

The mother of a seven-year-old boy, multiply handicapped by rubella, explained the reasons why other people would find her son difficult to care for:

> 'When he puts his fingers to his mouth it means he wants something to eat. Or cupping his hands means he wants a drink. People might not understand. And he gets sick a lot, and also has a lot of hospital appointments, so there would be too many interruptions really. . . . And his physical handicaps [a deformity of his Achilles tendon which meant he could not walk very well, plus bronchitis and croup and intermittent pneumonia] also mean he has lots of appointments. And when he comes

home from school he can't go out and play with the other children. He can't go out and do his own thing. It's pretty well constant attention, and we can't put on relatives too much.'

Since this woman was also very involved in teaching and stimulating her son, she found herself too tired to take on even a part-time job – especially in view of the difficulties of finding alternative care in the school holidays.

The difficulties of finding people willing to take on the responsibility of children with odd conditions or behaviour were described in great detail by the mother of a child with brittle bones, constantly in danger of fractures, by a woman whose daughter had a rare enzyme abnormality which meant that certain very common foods could make her very ill, and by the mother of a very handicapped spastic boy of eight, who said

'Normally I would be able to think of going full-time now, because when they come home from school you can find a friend or someone to take them in and look after them. Whereas nobody will look after Darren. Friends are all a bit nervous and frightened of handling him. They *like* him, but they just don't like to handle him. And if he holds his breath or anything like that, they just panic.'

This woman, whose husband was very poorly paid, was an outworker, doing sewing at home, but found that even the amount of sewing she could do was affected by her son's needs.

These depth interviews helped to make clear the processes by which disablement in children affected the paid employment of their mothers. The effect of the child's condition was complicated. It did not create a simple disjunction between being able or unable to go out to work. The majority of women interviewed were currently unable to work, though some had from time to time gone out to work. For those who were in paid employment at the time of the interview, caring for the child affected their working lives in a number of ways. They worked shorter hours or at different times of day, altered the type of work they did and so on. In the following section we see whether these views and experiences were echoed in the responses found when the whole sample of women with disabled children was asked about the child's effect on employment outside the home.

As Table 5.3 showed, 67 per cent of the women with disabled

children, as compared with 42 per cent of the women in the FES control group, were not in paid employment at the time of the study. More than half (57 per cent) of the women with disabled children not in paid employment attributed this to the child's condition, saying that had the child not been disabled they would now be in employment or actively seeking work. If these women had all, in fact, found jobs, the economic activity rate of the group would have been considerably higher than that of the control group – 76 per cent being economically active as opposed to 58 per cent of the women in the FES control. It is possible that this demonstrates only that hypothetical questions generate unrealistic answers. Hower it is also possible that these women's answers accurately reflect a heightened desire for employment outside the home among women with disabled children. Reasons for this increased desire would include both relief from stress and isolation and the wish to earn extra money to improve the quality of life of both the disabled child and the family. Previous studies of women with disabled children have stressed their desire for employment of some sort outside the home.[10]

It is also likely that some of the economically inactive women in the control group would have liked to go out to work but were unable to find jobs or to make suitable child-care arrangements.[11] Without comparable information on the numbers in the control who wanted but were unable to work, it is impossible to know whether the child's disability had in fact increased the desire for paid work in this sample of women with disabled children, or whether they were simply evincing an unsatisfied desire for paid employment shared by the general population of women with young children.

As noted above, 186 women (39 per cent of the sample) claimed that the child's disability prevented their going out to work at all at present. A further 25 said they were looking for work but had been unable to find a suitable job. Of these 211 women, 97 per cent said that their inability to work was caused because the child's disability restricted them in the ways described in Table 5.4. As this table indicates, many of them said they were affected for more than one reason.

As in the depth interviews, most women currently in paid employment reported that their working lives were affected by the child's condition. Of the 157 women in paid employment at the time of the survey, 121 (81 per cent) said that their employment

Table 5.4 Reasons why paid employment was not possible

Reasons (up to 3 recorded)	Frequency
Hours mother can work restricted to hours when child is in school	97
Frequent time off would be needed to cope with emergencies, etc.	65
Weeks mother can work restricted to weeks when child is in school (i.e. not school holidays)	53
Cannot work because child needs constant care by mother	39
Difficulties getting/does not want to get substitute care for child	37
Can only work in evenings	1
Cannot work/difficult to take work because of strain, sleepless nights, etc.	12
Can only work part-time (other than when child is in school or evenings)	10
Other answer	16
Total number of reasons	342
Total number of women giving at least one reason	204

was affected in a variety of ways. These were very similar to those mentioned above as preventing some women from working at all and, as there, many women cited several ways in which their work was affected. By far the commonest effect was adapting the mother's working hours so that one parent – usually the mother – was always at home when the disabled child was. For most women this was done by restricting their working hours to periods when the child was in school – i.e. working from around ten in the morning till two in the afternoon, often in term-time only. This meant taking jobs as school-meals attendants, barmaids, canteen and pensioners' lunch-club attendants and so on. Some women, however, were working twilight or evening shifts or doing early morning cleaning so that their husbands were at home while they were at work. Some women worked night shifts – as nursing auxiliaries, for example. The mother of a ten-year-old boy with spina bifida could not work during the day because the local school for normal children would accept her son as a pupil only on condition that she was always available to manage his incontinence. She worked evening shifts in a textile mill locally, which she minded very much because she missed being at home at bed-time to put her child to bed:

'I don't believe mothers should go out at night. . . . I believe I've missed out, because it's a pleasure bed-timing them. I would much rather go out 9 while 3 and be home evenings.'

Apart from restricting their actual hours, the next commonest effect mentioned was having to take time off when children were ill or for hospital appointments. One hundred and four women (70 per cent of those in employment) said they sometimes had to take time off work on such occasions; 23 women said they needed *frequent* time off. Of the women who sometimes had to take time off work, 76 per cent lost money whenever this happened.

Another effect claimed by a sizeable group of women – 34 per cent of those who were in paid employment – was taking jobs below the level of their qualifications or experience. These were women in casual or part-time work who had some training or experience they were unable to utilize at present, such as commercial or secretarial experience or hairdressing and similar skills. Ten women were qualified teachers or nurses but were currently doing unskilled work as clerical workers, home helps, school-dinner attendants and barmaids. The depth interviews showed that both the frustration and the financial losses of women in this position could be considerable. For example, the mother of a fourteen-year-old hyperactive boy had had to give up a responsible and well paid job as a supervisor for a cleaning firm and instead did evening and early morning cleaning jobs. A woman whose five-year-old daughter had Still's disease had tried to go back to nursing, for which she was trained, in the year before the study. For a time she managed, by doing constant night duty, but had had to give up because both parents felt their family life was suffering. Another woman, whose twelve-year-old daughter had Down's syndrome together with a heart defect and chronic bronchitis, had similarly had to abandon her nursing career. At the time of the study she was working in an antique shop but felt that she would soon have to give that up, since her frequent time off meant that the shop often had to close. A woman who had previously worked as a highly paid statistics clerk with the Midlands Electricity Board and whose cerebral-palsied fifteen-year-old son was extremely disabled was now working three evenings a week as a barmaid.

For some of the women in the study this change in the level of their work might have happened anyway. Recent studies of the employment patterns of married women[12] delineate a fairly typical pattern of employment in skilled non-manual jobs before the birth of children, followed by an initial return to the labour market in less skilled, often manual, part-time work. However, there is clear evidence from this study that women with disabled children are financially disadvantaged in relation to their peer groups. Of the women who said their work was affected in any way, 85 per cent claimed that this reduced their earnings; the comparative data corroborates this claim. These women had a much smaller chance, than the general population of women with older children especially, of breaking out of part-time casual and unskilled work, of resuming former careers or of training for new ones. The depth interviews showed how frustrating this could be. The mother of a totally dependent quadriplegic boy who had no speech but was of above average intelligence, for example, had always wanted to be a nursery nurse but had been unable to train because her son's care was so demanding. Having done voluntary work in a local nursery for five years she was, at the time of the survey, employed part-time there as a lunch-time helper with still no prospect of becoming professionally qualified.

The subjective information from the survey and from the depth interviews reflected the varied ways in which individual women responded to their child's disability. However, even in the depth interviews, certain themes recurred sufficiently often to suggest that they had more than individual validity. One was the increasing desire of women whose children were growing older to work outside the home – and their frustration as they became aware how a job could benefit both themselves and their families. Another was that finding employment typically involved a search for the *ideal* job with the right hours, school holidays off and understanding employers who did not mind regular days away. Finding such jobs could take a long time – one woman had waited four years for a job as a school-meals attendant. When for some reason the job came to an end, it could be extremely difficult to find another. Finding and staying in work could mean restructuring working hours and parenting responsibilities and some loss of shared time for parents themselves.

A third theme to emerge was that for many women, and particularly when their children were young, the terms 'working' and 'not working' did not accurately reflect their relationship to the labour market. Rather than being committed to working or staying at home they were in and out of employment – spending sometimes long and sometimes shorter periods at work. This, as other studies have pointed out,[13] is generally true of women with children – at least until their children become fairly independent. Disablement in a child accentuates this general tendency in three ways. First, since their dependency persists, this unstable relationship to employment lasts longer when a child is disabled. Second, the child's disablement itself is a reason for jobs being given up because they do not fit in with the disabled child's needs. New jobs, taken on experimentally, had been abandoned quite frequently by the women in the follow-up interviews. Finally, whereas mothers of normal children, not yet ready to enter the labour market permanently, can work for a spell to help the family through a financial crisis, to save for a new car or washing machine, for Christmas or for holidays, the mothers in our sample were acutely aware that they did not have the choice of working for a spell in this way. Women whose husbands had been made redundant or were facing redundancy, who had lost their jobs for other reasons or whose businesses were going badly regretted their inability to help out. Others mentioned being unable to work for a spell to help when there were big bills to pay or when, for whatever reason, they were short of money. The mother of a twelve-year-old girl with cystic fibrosis, for example, who was unable to go to school, had been unable to take a job in a local textile mill to help out when, because her husband was on short time, they got into arrears with mortgage, fuel and telephone bills.

It is often assumed that the impact of disablement increases with its severity. The truth of this assumption was tested in relation both to women's and to men's employment. Was it, that is, the severity of the child's condition that critically influenced whether parents went out to work and their hours of work? Or were particular types of disability such as incontinence or behaviour problems more important obstacles?

In the case of women a strong relationship was found between the severity of the child's condition and women's employment patterns. As the severity of the condition increased both labour-force participation and hours of work decreased. However the disabled child's age was also an important factor. As she grew older women's labour-force participation increased, even though the condition had not improved. Presumably it becomes easier to arrange alternative care as the child's condition becomes more predictable and the other children in the family become more independent. Women with a disabled child are also likely to share what is increasingly the normal expectation of women that they will resume work outside the home as children grow older.

Some types of impairment did appear more likely than others to influence women to stay at home. The mothers of children with very impaired mobility or severe difficulties in communication, those who regularly experienced severe pain or who had frequent fits were significantly less likely to work outside their homes than women whose disabled children did not have these problems. It is understandable that parents whose children are in pain or are unable to communicate their basic needs to strangers may be less willing or less able to leave them with unfamiliar people. This finding has implications for the planning of acceptable forms of alternative care for such children, suggesting that one-to-one forms of care rather than group care may be required.

There was clear evidence, then, that severe disablement in a child was associated with striking differences in the employment patterns and earnings of women, that these differences became more marked as children grew up and that the severity and type of disability influenced women's employment patterns. In the following section the employment patterns and earnings of men are examined to see whether they were similarly affected.

The work and earnings of men with disabled children

Remarkably little is known about the ways in which fatherhood typically affects men's work and earnings.[14] Ignorance of the effect of fatherhood *per se* inevitably affects our ability to judge the reliability of the subjective accounts men with disabled children give of the child's effect on their working lives. Their experience may be common to most men with children. Previous studies have, nevertheless, found substantial numbers of men with a disabled child claiming that the child's needs affected their working lives in a variety of ways. One study by the Family Fund research team, for example, found 25 per cent of men with a disabled child claiming that their work had been affected. Smaller-scale studies corroborate this finding.[15] The commonest effect cited is a reduction in earnings. However in most studies a small minority of men also report that the child's disablement has caused them to *increase* their earnings.

It is credible that severe disablement in a child may restrict the earning capacity of fathers as well as of mothers. Some children will be too dependent for mothers to manage continuously without help and men will therefore be needed at home – both to give their wives a break and, for example, to help escort children to hospital appointments. Some men may lose promotion because they choose not to move away from specialist facilities or supportive family and neighbourhood networks. Others may not achieve their potential because the child's special needs mean that they are unable (or unwilling) to pursue their careers as single-mindedly as they would otherwise have done.

It seems equally possible, however, that men may respond to severe disablement in a child by *increasing* their working hours and earnings. Given the lower earning capacity of women it may appear sensible, financially at least, for the work of caring and earning to be divided between parents so that the former falls completely to women and the latter to men. On this reading men would seek to increase their earnings, both to compensate for the loss of a wife's earnings and to provide for expenses arising from the child's condition.

In the following section, two kinds of data are examined to see which of these responses appeared to be more common among this sample of men with a disabled child: first, the accounts of the men with disabled children themselves and, second, comparative data on the participation rates and earnings of the men with disabled children and the FES control.[16]

Subjective views of the child's effect on men's working lives

The great majority of the men in this sample – 77 per cent – reported that their working lives had been affected by the child's condition in at least one way. The commonest effects mentioned were on the kind of job done, on working hours and time away from work, and on promotion prospects. For a very small group of men the child's condition had led directly to job loss.

Job changes

Fifteen per cent of the men in the sample reported having changed their jobs at least once as a result of the child's condition. The commonest reasons given for changing jobs were, first, a desire for more flexibility or a reduction in working hours, and second, dissatisfaction with jobs which took men away from home. Implicit in these reasons was a desire to be more available to help with the disabled child's care or simply be more involved in her upbringing. However reasons other than sharing in the child's care were also given. A small number of men mentioned changing to jobs which were better paid, because of the child's expenses and their wives' inability to go out to work. One man, with a thirteen-year-old cerebral-palsied child, had given up his job solely in order to claim back his superannuation as a lump sum, this being the only way he could replace the family's car. Four men said they had changed jobs to work in places where there was more suitable housing or to be near better services.

Overtime

Eighty-two men (18 per cent of those currently in employment) said that the child's condition affected the amount of overtime they worked. Sixty-seven (15 per cent) said they were able to do less overtime, while fifteen (3 per cent) said they worked extra overtime because the child's disablement meant they needed more money.

Time off work

Three hundred and two men (68 per cent) said they regularly had to take time off work because of the child's condition, the most frequent reason given being the need to escort the child to medical appointments of various sorts. Looking after the child when she was ill or difficult or when a mother herself was ill was also fairly common. Just over half of those who took time off work in this way lost money when they did. This overall figure conceals considerable differences between non-manual and manual workers: 60 per cent of manual, as against 16 per cent of non-manual, workers lost money when they took time off.

Losing jobs

Unskilled manual workers appeared to be at risk of losing jobs when they took too much time off work. One man, for example, who was only nineteen when his first child was born severely disabled by spina bifida, lost a lot of time from his job as a packer in the year after her birth, when she was frequently in hospital and had several major operations. He was dismissed when his daughter was re-admitted to hospital and he once again took time off to visit her. Another man lost his job as a van driver when he had to take time off to look after his wife who had had a third breakdown under the stress of caring for their totally dependent quadriplegic son and two other small children.

Damage to promotion prospects

Eighty-six men (20 per cent) said that the child's condition had limited their chances of promotion. These were predominantly men in professional and managerial occupations and the commonest reasons for their failure to achieve promotion were their inability to move around and the need for frequent time away from work. The depth interviews provided abundant illustration of the ways in which men were held back and their responses to this. The father of a deaf child, for example, explained the effect of his child's disablement on his career:

> 'The principal problem is [that] I work for a national company, which means opportunities for promotion or whatever would come about quicker, perhaps, if I was prepared to move about the country. But the situation has been, with Ann, that we felt that the help and training we've had here has been so good, that we obviously don't want to break up the start of a relationship with her teacher which is obviously of benefit to her. So when I am – as I have been – offered other positions (I was offered one in Leicester which offered more money and more prospects and was more satisfying in that way) I decided, purely on account of Ann, not to move. . . . And at the moment, while I'm waiting for the next position, I'm losing up to £2,000 a year. . . . Family and home have a high priority to me anyway, and that makes you make judgments about how much time you devote to your work, and all that sort of thing, but the problem is more sharply defined because of Ann, because it just adds to it and becomes more important because of her and the pressures she puts on my wife. So I may well not put as much time into my job as I would otherwise do, and this affects my earnings. My company does pay on performance. If you do a good job they recognize it in

Incomes 89

terms of cash. . . . But if I was prepared, say, to take clients out in the evening, entertain them, then I could probably achieve more with them . . . which could make me earn even more money.'

Not all men are willing to sacrifice their career prospects. An interesting counter-example was provided by an extremely successful architect who had never at any time allowed his daughter's disablement (she was by then ten, with Down's syndrome, a serious heart defect and chronic bronchitis) to affect his career. His wife was herself a qualified nurse who wanted, but was unable, to pursue her own career and was very resentful of her husband's attitude. At the time of the interview this couple had just decided to separate.

Comparative data

Comparison with FES data allowed us to investigate the extent to which these effects on men's working lives were reflected in their working hours and earnings (see Table 5.5). This data was limited in one important respect. It related only to the jobs men held at the time of the study and did not allow longer-term effects on occupational choices or earnings to be assessed. Whether these men might have been in different occupations or promoted to higher grades had their child not been disabled therefore remains unknown. The occupational structure of the two samples was different, more of the men with a disabled child than of men in the control being in manual occupations. However lack of reliable information on the general population of children with disabilities means that we cannot say whether this difference reflects class differences in the incidence of disablement, effects on men's occupational choices, or bias in the sampling frame from which the families with a disabled child were drawn.[17]

Labour-force participation

Only among unskilled manual workers were noticeable differences in participation rates found. Table 5.5 shows that 24 per cent of unskilled manual workers with disabled children as compared with 10 per cent of unskilled manual workers in the control were unemployed at the time of the study. The number of men involved is probably too small to support firm conclusions about the increased risk of unemployment among men with a disabled child. The survey of families with a disabled child did, however, show how disablement could precipitate unemployment among men. There were seven men in the sample who were unemployed and who attributed that directly to their child's disablement. All seven were manual workers. One gave his own ill-health as the reason for not being in work, his unemployment arising from stomach ulcers caused, he said, by worrying about his son who was seven, with a severe congenital abnormality of bowel and bladder. The remaining six said they had been forced to give up work mainly because their wives could no longer cope unaided with the disabled child and all their other family responsibilities. All these children posed severe management problems. One was a boy of fifteen, over six feet tall, and heavy, who was severely mentally handicapped and subject to *grand mal* epileptic fits. Another was a severely mentally handicapped girl of seven who was hyperactive, incontinent and totally without speech. She attended school only one and a half days of the week, and there were two other children of twelve and fourteen in the family. Of the remaining two men, one had previously worked away, as an electrician's mate on contract jobs. His wife needed him to be nearer home to help when she could not manage. The last man had given up his job essentially as part of a strategy to get more suitable housing. He was on a government retraining scheme, linked to a job in a new town where they would be able to afford (as they could not in London where they were currently living) a house with a garden which would help the family cope with their hyperactive ten-year-old and improve the quality of his life, too.

Earnings and hours of work

On average, the men with a disabled child earned £8.70 a week less than the men in the control. However, the different occupational structures of the two samples meant that it was necessary to look separately at the earnings of non-manual and manual workers and of men in similar occupation groups (see Table 5.5).

This revealed considerable differences between non-manual and manual workers with disabled children. In general the earnings of manual workers with a disabled child were very similar to those of

Incomes 91

Table 5.5 Men's paid employment

	Participation* rate (%)		Mean weekly† hours		Mean weekly† earnings (£)		Number of employed men	
	Families with a disabled child	Control group	Families with a disabled child	Control group	Families with a disabled child	Control group	Families with a disabled child	Control group
All employees	92	95	44	44	83.3	92.0	403	605
Non-manual employees	98	99	40	42	90.9	108.9	98	232
Manual employees	93	94	45	45	80.9	81.4	305	366
Occupation group:								
Professional/technical	100	99	38	42	98.6	105.1	24	86
Administrative/managerial	100	99	44	43	82.9	124.0	31	86
Teachers	100	100	39	38	94.5	101.3	8	26
Clerical workers	94	97	39	42	94.8	87.8	32	30
Shop workers	100	100	41	39	60.4	76.9	3	4
Skilled manual workers	95	96	45	45	84.1	83.3	189	235
Semi-skilled manual workers	93	90	46	45	76.7	77.9	100	113
Unskilled manual workers	76	90	44	48	69.9	78.9	16	18

Base: All non self-employed men.
*Participating men are defined as those employed in the survey period.
†Calculations are based only on those employees for whom information on both hours and earnings was recorded in the survey period.

manual workers in the FES. Non-manual workers with a disabled child, on the other hand, earned substantially less than their FES counterparts – on average £18 a week. This general pattern broke down at the level of individual occupation groups, however. One group of non-manual workers with a disabled child – clerical workers – had higher earnings than clerical workers in the FES; one group of manual workers with a disabled child – unskilled manual workers – had lower earnings than FES men in similar occupations.

The average 'gap' of £18 a week among men in non-manual occupations also concealed variations in the size of the earnings difference in different occupation groups. Administrative and managerial workers, for example, earned £41.10 a week less, on average, than FES men in similar occupations. The difference for the other non-manual occupation groups was less than half this amount. Unskilled manual workers with a disabled child earned an average of £9 a week less than their FES counterparts. Given the much lower level of their earnings the impact of such a loss must have been if anything greater than for the higher-earning non-manual workers.

It would appear then that, in general, disablement in a child is more likely to cause earnings loss among men in non-manual than in manual occupations. However the earnings figures presented here are based on men's *normal* earnings.[18] They do not reflect intermittent earnings loss, to which manual workers are particularly vulnerable. The true effect of a child's disablement on the earnings of manual workers is likely, in consequence, to be underestimated by these figures.

Interestingly, the lower earnings of the men with disabled children were not caused by their working much shorter hours than the men in the FES control. With the exception of unskilled manual workers, who did work much shorter hours than their FES counterparts and also earned much less, the men with disabled children in the other occupation groups were working slightly *longer* hours for similar or smaller amounts of money (see Table 5.5).

This information on hours is not reliable for non-manual work, where the hours formally required can often be a poor guide to the time devoted to work. In the case of manual workers it would appear that, apart from occasional time off, disablement in a child did not have a marked effect on the hours worked by the majority.

Nor did it cause them to do less overtime. Indeed slightly more of the manual workers with disabled children did overtime – 44 per cent as against 32 per cent of the FES control – while those who did overtime worked virtually the same number of overtime hours.

It was suggested earlier that severe disablement in a child might cause men either to increase their earnings to offset loss of earnings by their wives or, alternatively, to reduce their work commitments in order to help with the disabled child's care, thereby suffering earnings loss.

This study provided no support for the suggestion that disablement in a child typically leads men to increase their earnings. On the contrary, both the subjective accounts of the men themselves and comparative data on their earnings suggested that the working lives of most men with disabled children and the earnings of many were adversely affected.

The picture that emerged from the comparative earnings data was not, however, of a clear-cut loss of earnings by most men with a disabled child. Nor was there any evidence, as there had been for women, that earnings loss rose with the severity of the condition. On the contrary, men's earnings appeared to rise as the severity of the child's condition increased.[19]

Taking the samples as a whole, the earnings of the men with disabled children were an average of £8.70 a week less than those of men in the control. However this average conceals a patchy picture. The disabled child's effect on men's earnings varied both between men in non-manual and manual occupations and between men in different occupation groups. The comparative findings on men's earnings were less consistent, then, than for women's.

This lack of consistency must, in part, reflect real variations in the impact of a child's disablement on men's working lives. At the most basic level, men vary in their willingness to become involved in domestic tasks at the expense of their own working lives. Child care is conventionally viewed as a female role. It cannot be assumed that disablement in a child will necessarily alter the domestic division of labour – particularly when women's lower earnings potential can make it appear sensible for men to concentrate on supporting the family financially while women take responsibility for running the home and caring for children.[20]

Even when men *are* willing to become involved in the disabled child's care their ability to do so, and the extent to which this is translated into earnings loss will vary both with the type of employment they are in and the attitudes of employers. Some jobs are flexible, allowing men to be at home when needed without loss of earnings. Others are much less so and men are free to help at home only by taking time off. Employers, too, vary in their responses to men's needs for time off. Some are extremely generous. Others, as we have seen, dismiss men when too much time off is taken. In general, non-manual occupations appeared to offer the men in this study more freedom to help at home. Men in manual occupations were less free to rearrange their working hours so as to help with the child and tended to take time off instead, losing money when they did so. As we have seen, the earnings lost as a result of sporadic time off could not be identified in this study. Almost certainly, therefore, the impact of disablement in a child on the earnings of men in manual occupations has been underestimated.

Restricting comparisons, as we have done, to men in similar occupations at the time of the study is also likely to mean that the disabled child's effect on men's careers and earnings in the longer term has been underestimated. Our interviews with the fathers of disabled children pointed to substantial effects on their careers – both among professional men whose promotion prospects were damaged and among manual workers who frequently mentioned taking less lucrative jobs which did not take them away from home. The extent of such effects cannot, unfortunately, be tested from the present study.

Clearly, in order to measure the effect of a child's disablement on men's occupational choices and earnings with complete accuracy, more information is needed. This should not be allowed to obscure the present study's finding that disablement in a child was associated with lower earnings by men. When differences in the two groups' occupational structures had been taken into account, the earnings of the men with disabled children remained £8 a week less, on average, than those of men in the FES control.[21] Fuller information would almost certainly demonstrate that the true gap is considerably wider.

Income from social security

The cash benefits paid on account of disablement are an important source of extra income for families with a disabled child. As we saw earlier, social security payments formed a much higher proportion of income for the families with disabled children than for the control families – 19 per cent as against 5 per cent (see Table 5.2). The difference in these proportions is almost entirely due to the benefits paid on account of the child's disablement, that is attendance and mobility allowances. A maximum of £21 a week was available from these benefits at the time of this study: £14 for the higher-rate attendance allowance and £7 for mobility allowance.

It is often assumed, in talking about the cash help available to families with severely disabled children, that most of them receive the maximum amount available. This is not so. The average amount received in disability benefits by this sample of families with a disabled child was £14 a week, as compared with the theoretical maximum of £21. The numbers of families receiving different benefit 'packages' and the impact of these benefits on families' incomes is examined below. Before this, however, we look briefly at the purposes of these benefits and at their take-up among the study families.

Attendance allowance

Attendance allowance is a benefit paid to disabled people who require a substantial amount of care of supervision. In the case of disabled children it is paid only to children over two, and the attendance or supervision required must be substantially in excess of that required by a child of the same age or sex. The allowance is paid at two rates, according to whether the extra care or supervision is needed both in the daytime and during the night, or in only one of these periods. As Table 5.6 shows, 95 per cent of the families with disabled children in this study were receiving attendance allowances, 53 per cent of them at the higher rate (then £14 a week) and 42 per cent at the lower rate (then £9.30 a week).

The purpose of attendance allowance is not entirely clear. The original intention in introducing it was simply to direct some extra financial help to very severely disabled people. What this extra financial help was *for* was not clear. It was certainly not primarily meant to compensate for earnings lost by carers. If a purpose for attendance allowance can be identified at all, this was to help with the costs, in the widest sense, of severe disablement. The different elements in these costs – higher day-to-day living costs, the need to buy services, and earnings loss by carers – were not distinguished.

Confusion arises from the disjunction between this unspecific, compensatory, purpose and the criteria adopted to embody it. Attendance needs were chosen as a way of identifying the people who were most severely disabled, and hence in greatest need of help. However this emphasis on attendance creates a tendency for attendance allowance to be regarded, mistakenly, as compensation for earnings lost by carers. This is particularly true in the case of disabled children where the main carer is usually the child's mother and the allowance paid to her. Hence it can happen that the attendance allowance is viewed both as compensation for women's lost earnings and as help with the extra costs of disablement. It is certainly not generous enough to do both. Clearly, however, in the absence of a more rational basis for disability benefits, in which extra costs and carers' earnings losses are separately recognized, confusion about the purpose of attendance allowance will persist.

Mobility allowance

The purpose of mobility allowance is entirely clear.[22] It is a benefit designed to help with the higher transport costs of people unable or virtually unable to walk because of physical disablement and likely to remain so for at least a year. The weekly value of mobility allowance at the time of the study was £7. As the criteria indicate, the coverage of the mobility allowance is more restricted than that of attendance allowance, and this is reflected in the much smaller number of children in this sample receiving the benefit: 37 per cent

Table 5.6 Disability benefits received

Benefit	No. of families		% of families	
Attendance allowance	458		95	
- higher-rate		256		53
- lower rate		202		42
Mobility allowance	180		37	
No benefits received	21		4	
Total number of families		480		

of them received mobility allowance, as against the 95 per cent who had attendance allowances (see Table 5.6).

The value of the benefits received

The amounts the families with disabled children were receiving in disability benefits varied greatly. Only 27 per cent of the families in this sample were receiving the maximum possible amount of £21.00 a week; at the other end of the scale 4 per cent received nothing at all (see Table 5.7).

Table 5.7 Benefits received and their value

Benefits received	No.	%
Higher-rate attendance + mobility allowance (£21.00 p.w.)	127	27
Lower-rate attendance + mobility allowance (£16.30 p.w.)	51	11
Higher-rate attendance allowance only (£14.00 p.w.)	129	27
Lower-rate attendance allowance only (£9.30 p.w.)	151	32
Mobility allowance only (£7.00 p.w.)	1	–
No disability benefits	21	4
Total	480	

Table 5.8 shows the importance of the benefit 'package' received in closing the gap between the incomes of the families with a disabled child and those of the control families. Only where families were receiving the maximum possible amount of £21 a week were their incomes slightly higher than those of the FES families; the average incomes of the families receiving no disability benefits at all were £19.50 a week less.

Table 5.8 raises interesting questions about the equity of the criteria on which benefits are currently allocated, particularly in relation to children who received higher-rate attendance but not mobility allowances. These children's families were considerably worse off than those of children who received mobility allowance in addition to their higher-rate attendance allowances. However the children themselves were no less severely disabled than those who received both higher-rate attendance and mobility allowances. Moreover they were significantly *more* disabled than children who received lower-rate attendance allowances and mobility allowances – worth £2.30 a week more.[23]

A much higher proportion of the families receiving only higher-

Table 5.8 Family income by benefits received

Benefits received		Mean gross income £ per week	No.
Higher-rate attendance + mobility allowance	(£21.00 p.w.)	118.3	109
Lower-rate attendance + mobility allowance	(£16.30 p.w.)	116.2	47
Higher-rate attendance allowance only	(£14.00 p.w.)	108.8	119
Lower-rate attendance allowance only	(£9.30 p.w.)	105.5	143
Mobility allowance only	(£7.00 p.w.)	98.3	1
No disability benefits		97.2	19
Control group		116.7	640

rate attendance allowances than of those receiving only lower-rate attendance allowances fell into the lowest income ranges: 22 per cent of the former as against 13 per cent of the latter having incomes of less than £80 per week. This presumably reflects the fact that the children who qualified for higher-rate attendance allowances were more severely disabled and less likely, therefore, to have mothers in paid employment. These children suffer a financial disadvantage because, though very severely disabled, they are not eligible for mobility allowance, which is based on the presence of a particular type of impairment rather than on the overall severity of a child's condition or its dependence on others. Had extra financial help been given to the most severely disabled children on the basis of severity of disability or handicap rather than on the presence of locomotor impairment, this would have avoided their apparently inequitable treatment *vis-à-vis* those children receiving mobility allowances in addition to attendance allowances. However the question of whether it is equitable to pay different rates of benefit to people who are equally disabled depends on the purpose of benefits and their criteria and the relation of both of these to need. Since attendance and mobility allowances are separate benefits with different purposes and criteria it might not be considered legitimate to consider them together as a disability income expected to bear some relation to severity of disablement and, hence, to need.

Mobility allowance was designed to help with the higher transport costs assumed to arise from severe locomotor impairment. If people with such impairments do have higher transport costs than others whose overall disablement is equally severe, it may be equitable to pay mobility allowances to those who have them (except in as much as other costs are not similarly recognized). However, it has frequently been claimed that the mobility allowance criteria do not identify the children with the highest transport costs.[24] The Pearson Commission decided that they did not, and recommended extending the criteria to include children over two, with a wider range of disabilities.[25] The analysis of transport expenditure data in the present study points to a similar conclusion.[26] Clearly, then, the basis on which mobility allowance in particular is awarded warrants further scrutiny.

The overall effect on incomes

So far, earnings and disability benefits have been considered in isolation. The question that arises naturally at this point is what, at the end of the day, was the overall effect of the child's condition on families' incomes? A complete answer to that question would have to take into account both parental earnings loss and any extra costs arising from the child's condition, balancing these against the value of the disability benefits received. For the moment, however, we are concerned only with the money coming in. How it is spent is the subject of the next chapter.

The question then arises of whether disability benefits should be included in income. Since they are largely intended to help with the special needs arising from disablement they might justifiably be excluded from family income. However disability benefits are not invariably kept separate and used exclusively for the disabled child's special needs.[27] They are therefore counted here as part of family income. Clearly, however, having once been included in income disability benefits cannot be assumed to be available to help with these special needs.

As was noted earlier, the different proportions of non-manual and manual workers in the two samples made it necessary to compare the incomes of families with heads in non-manual and manual occupations separately. This revealed that the effect of the child's disablement varied greatly with income. In general the richer, non-manual, families with disabled children were substantially poorer than their FES counterparts; manual families, on the other hand, were slightly better off.[28] The gross incomes of the former were an average of £15.50 a week less than those of similar FES families; those of the latter £4.30 a week more. Disablement in a child seemed, that is, to prevent families from being either as poor or as prosperous as they might otherwise have been.

The effect of the child's disablement on family income was also found to vary considerably with the age of the youngest child in the family. For both non-manual and manual families in the control group income increased steadily with the age of the youngest child (see Figure 5.1). This steady progress was not found among the families with disabled children.

Among the non-manual families with disabled children family income actually fell as children grew up: the median income of the families whose youngest child was eleven or over was lower than that of families whose youngest child was under five. Differences

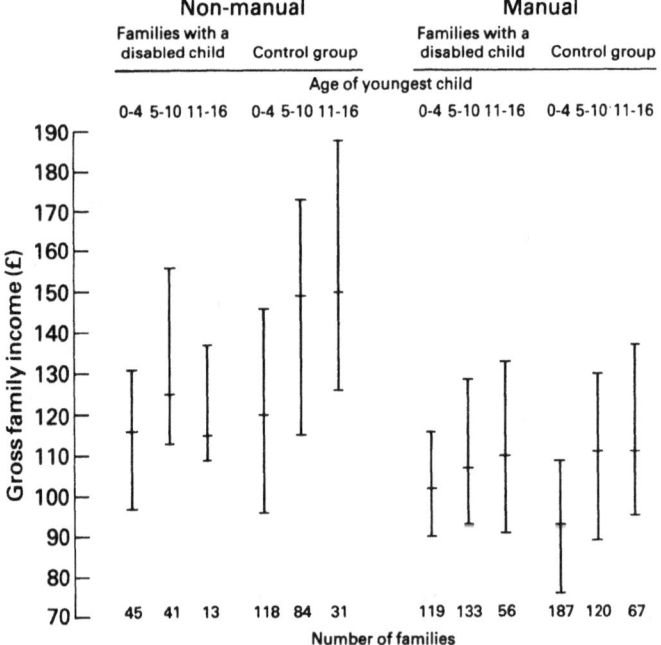

Figure 5.1 Median and interquartile range of gross family income by family type

between these families' incomes and those of the non-manual families in the control were large and increased dramatically as children grew up – from a difference of £11.00 a week in average incomes when the youngest child in the family was under five to a difference of £46.40 when the youngest child was eleven or over.

Among manual families the differences were smaller and the life-cycle effect of the child's disablement very different. The financial 'advantage' of the manual families with a disabled child was found to be confined to families whose youngest child was under five. Their incomes were £9.50 a week higher, on average, than those of similar FES families. The higher incomes of the families with disabled children at this stage presumably reflect their receipt of attendance allowances at a stage when relatively few women in the control had earnings. As children grew older and more women in the control went out to work this financial advantage was gradually lost. By the time the youngest child in the family was eleven or over the manual families with a disabled child were an average of £3.00 a week worse off than similar families in the control.

At the end of the day, then, even when disability benefits were included in income, substantial differences remained between the incomes of the families with disabled children and those of the control families. Only for manual workers whose youngest child was under five did disability benefits close the income gap between the families with disabled children and the control, leaving a margin to help with the disabled child's special needs. They made particularly little impression on the much higher earnings losses experienced by virtually all non-manual families – particularly as children grew up and the combined earnings losses of men and women increasingly excluded families with a disabled child from the prosperity experienced at that stage by their peers.

Disposable incomes

The comparisons made so far have related to families' gross incomes. Differences in command over resources are reflected more clearly, however, in what families finally have to spend after the redistribution of income via taxes and benefits. We therefore conclude this chapter by comparing the two samples' disposable incomes. The effect of deducting disability benefits from income, and hence clarifying the impact of the child's disablement on parental earnings, is also shown.

Differences in disposable incomes closely mirrored the pattern that had emerged from comparing their gross incomes, though since the distribution of disposable incomes is narrower the differences between them were smaller. Taking the samples as a whole, the average disposable incomes of the families with a disabled child were £3.40 a week smaller than those of the control families. As with gross incomes this average deficit concealed a difference in the effect on richer and poorer families. The disposable income of the non-manual families was, on average, £8.30 a week less than that of similar control families; that of manual families £3.77 a week more.

The value of a family's income depends on the number of people to be supported and, in the case of children, their ages. Hence incomes data are not strictly comparable unless the families whose incomes are being compared are identical in these respects or the data adjusted to take account of any differences. This can be done in a number of ways. The method adopted for the present study, where the numbers and ages of the children in the two samples were not identical, was to express each family's disposable income as a proportion of its supplementary benefit entitlement. Supplementary benefit scales increase as children get older, reflecting their greater needs. They therefore provide a convenient way of standardizing incomes to remove the effect of differences in family composition.[29]

Taking account of differences in family composition in this way confirmed the picture that had previously emerged (see Table 5.9). When disability benefits were included in income poor families with disabled children were less likely to be poor and richer families less likely to be as rich as similar families in the control.

As we have seen, the financial advantage of the poorer families with disabled children is caused by disability benefits. However neither attendance nor mobility allowances would be included in families' resources in calculating entitlement to supplementary benefit. To compare the two groups' disposable incomes from the perspective of the supplementary benefits scheme – their incomes 'relative to need' – disability benefits should be deducted from income. Doing so completely removes the financial advantage of the poorer families with disabled children, leaving many more of them than of the control families in the lowest income band (see Table 5.9).

Table 5.9 Disposable incomes relative to need

	Families with a disabled child		Control group
Percentage of supplementary benefit level	Including all disability benefits % of families	Net of disability benefits % of families	% of families
Non-manual families			
80– 99	0.0	0.0	0.4
100–139	1.0	7.0	1.3
140–199	17.0	36.0	15.7
200–300	61.0	47.0	45.6
over 300	21.0	10.0	37.0
Manual families			
80– 99	0.0	1.8	1.0
100–139	3.6	18.2	8.0
140–199	29.5	43.8	28.2
200–300	56.0	31.0	49.5
over 300	10.9	5.2	13.4

Differences in disposable incomes in real money terms are shown in Table 5.10. Here, as before, the effect of disablement on income varies with occupational status and with the age of the family's youngest child. When disability benefits are included in income non-manual families with a disabled child invariably have smaller incomes than similar control families, the gap widening as children grow up and reaching its maximum of £30.30 a week when the youngest child in the family is over eleven. The poorer, manual, families are better off when their youngest child is under five but progressively lose ground after that. By the time the youngest child is over eleven their disposable incomes are an average of £2.20 a week less than those of manual families in the control. To take account of increases in earnings and benefits between 1978 and 1984 the figures in Table 5.10 (like the other figures in this chapter) should, roughly, be doubled. On this basis the disposable incomes of non-manual families with disabled children whose children were all over eleven would have been in the region of £60 a week less than the incomes of similar families in the control in 1984.[30]

Deducting disability benefits from disposable incomes allows the impact of the child's condition on parental earnings at different stages of the family life-cycle to emerge. As Table 5.10 shows, income from sources other than disability benefits is invariably lower among the families with disabled children, and the difference increases markedly as children grow up.

The effectiveness of existing benefits in mitigating earnings loss depends, clearly, on the amount lost. For manual workers whose youngest child is under five an original earnings deficit of £6.40 a week was translated into an advantage of £5.90 a week over similar FES families. For non-manual families whose youngest child was over eleven an original earnings deficit of £48 a week was narrowed only to £30.30 (see Table 5.10).

As already observed, existing disability benefits are not in any case intended to compensate for parental earnings loss. That such wide discrepancies remain when they are included in income indicates the need for a benefit which would explicitly recognize

Table 5.10 Real disposable incomes

	Families with a disabled child Mean £ per week	Control group Mean £ per week
Non-manual families		
Youngest child under 5		
Including disability benefits	96.3	
Net of disability benefits	84.7	103.2
Youngest child 5–10		
Including disability benefits	114.4	
Net of disability benefits	100.0	119.5
Youngest child 11–16		
Including disability benefits	102.7	
Net of disability benefits	85.0	133.0
Manual families		
Youngest child under 5		
Including disability benefits	83.4	
Net of disability benefits	71.1	77.5
Youngest child 5–10		
Including disability benefits	92.1	
Net of disability benefits	77.5	91.6
Youngest child 11–16		
Including disability benefits	91.1	
Net of disability benefits	76.0	93.3

earnings loss among parents with disabled children. The case for such a benefit is discussed further in the concluding chapter of this book.

Summary

The incomes of this sample of families with a severely disabled child were found to be lower, on average, than those of the control families even when benefits intended to help with the costs of disablement were included in their incomes. Their lower incomes were caused by differences in the employment patterns and earnings of both parents. Differences in women's participation rates and earnings were particularly marked, the women with a disabled child being much less likely to go out to work and, when they did, to work fewer hours and earn less. This was true at all stages of the family life-cycle but was especially marked when the youngest child in the family was over eleven and the majority of women in the control in paid employment.

The picture in relation to men's earnings was less consistent. The earnings of men in most non-manual occupations who had a disabled child were appreciably less than those of similar FES men. There was reason to believe, moreover, that the study data understated the impact of the child's disablement on their earnings from loss of promotion or inability to change jobs. The majority of men in manual occupations appeared not to experience regular earnings loss. However the income data did not reflect sporadic earnings loss, which is likely to be experienced by manual workers with a disabled child. Overall, then, though there was clear evidence that the work and earnings of men with a disabled child were affected and their average earnings were less than those of the control, the results were less clear-cut than for women and almost certainly understated the true extent of earnings loss.

Disability benefits increased the incomes of the families with disabled children. However the amount received varied greatly and did not clearly relate to the severity of the child's condition. Only a quarter of the families with a disabled child received the theoretical maximum available; 4 per cent received no disability benefits at all.

The overall impact of the child's disablement depended on the family's income level. Up to a certain income level families with a disabled child were slightly better off than similar families in the control; beyond that point they were increasingly poorer. Thus, taking the samples as a whole, most families with a manual head were slightly richer than their FES counterparts and most non-manual families poorer. The effect on income also depended, however, on the ages of the children in the family. This is not, of course, independent of income. Most families are poorest when children are very young, becoming more prosperous as children grow up and parental earnings increase. Families with severely disabled children do not appear to experience this lifetime progression in their incomes. The incomes of the non-manual families with disabled children in this study in fact fell slightly as children grew up. Hence, though they were invariably poorer than similar families in the control the differences in their incomes increased dramatically as children grew up.

Among the poorer, mainly manual, families with disabled children the picture was somewhat different. Attendance allowances brought the incomes of families with a child under five above those of similar families in the control. After that stage their incomes increasingly fell behind those of the control, but the difference was much smaller than for non-manual families. In general, therefore, the effect of disablement in a child on family income was much greater for richer than poorer families and for families with older than younger children.

It is clear, then, that for the majority of families in this study the child's disablement meant that their incomes were lower than they would have been – even when benefits meant to help with the special expenses arising from disablement were taken into account. In the following chapter we investigate whether, in addition to its effect on their incomes, disablement in a child altered the way these families spent their money.

6 Expenditure

The costs of a child's disablement are not borne only by parents. They will be shared to some extent by other relatives, friends and neighbours and the community at large. Here, however, we are concerned with the costs which do fall to parents and with the extent to which these exceed those of bringing up any child.

Previous research has suggested that disablement in a child can affect family expenditure in a great many ways.[1] Extra spending may be needed on items bought regularly and which figure in all family budgets – food, fuel and clothing, for example. It may be for items which are bought much less frequently but which cost significant amounts of money – cars and other consumer durables, or specialized items such as wheelchairs or housing adaptations. There may also be episodes of expense which are difficult to foresee or plan for. Typical examples would be the need to move quickly to a more suitable house or to meet the costs which arise when a child is admitted to hospital.

Clearly, identifying the extent to which disablement creates costs beyond those normally encountered in child-raising will be complicated by the different time periods to which expenditure relates. That money may be spent on items not used by ordinary families or for contingencies they are unlikely to experience is an additional complication.

To overcome these complications as far as possible, three sources of information on the costs of disablement in a child were used in the present study:

1 Expenditure data from our replication of the FES together with comparable data for the control families.
2 Our survey of all the families with disabled children which asked parents about their own perceptions of the disabled child's costs.
3 Depth interviews with forty-eight of these families.

The information from the survey and depth interviews was obtained simply by asking parents to remember or estimate costs.

108 *Expenditure*

The FES, on the other hand, requires respondents to keep records of everything they spend over a two-week period.[2] From this we were able to compare the amounts spent by the two groups of families and hence to calculate the extra cost created by the child's disablement. However two weeks is too short a period to provide reliable information for items such as large consumer durables which are bought infrequently.[3] Neither can data of this sort tell us anything about episodes of financial stress arising from the condition, such as hospital admissions. To give a more complete picture the comparative expenditure data are therefore supplemented by information supplied by the parents of disabled children.

In the remainder of this chapter, then, the cost of disablement in a child is examined from three perspectives. First, the FES data are used to compare the amounts families in the two samples spent each week on a range of commodities. Larger, less regular purchases are then examined using subjective information from parents and comparative data on the ownership of certain assets. Finally, the costs associated with hospitals are illustrated from our depth interviews with parents.

Comparisons with the FES control

The FES classifies the vast range of items on which families spend their money into eleven main commodity groups and approximately a hundred sub-groups.[4] The majority of the expenditure figures presented here relate to the main FES commodity groups:

Food
Fuel, light and power
Clothing and footwear
Transport and vehicles
Alcoholic drink
Tobacco
Durable household goods
Services
Housing
{ Other goods
{ Miscellaneous goods[5]

These very broad categories can make it difficult to identify the effect of disablement on particular items. From time to time, therefore, expenditure on individual items within commodity groups is also compared.

As Chapter 5 showed, the incomes of the families with disabled children were different from those of the FES families. It was necessary to control for this so that any differences observed in expenditure did not simply reflect the fact that families in the two samples had different amounts to spend. This was done by grouping both samples into three broad ranges of disposable income and comparing the expenditures of families in each income range. The ranges of weekly disposable income chosen were: under £70; £70–£100; £100–£150.[6]

In the following section the average weekly expenditure of the families with disabled children on each of the main FES commodity groups is compared with that of the control families. Disabled children are not, however, a homogeneous group. The numbers of children said by parents to cause extra expense on different items varied greatly – from 32 per cent of the sample in the case of food to 83 per cent for cleaning materials. To calculate the extra costs of the families who *do* spend more on any item is difficult since there is no reliable way of identifying them. The somewhat rough and ready approach adopted here is to compare the expenditure of the families who reported that the child's condition caused extra expense on particular items with that of the control families.[7]

Food

Disablement can affect a child's eating pattern in a number of different ways. Conditions such as cystic fibrosis and diabetes, for example, mean that some normal foods cannot be tolerated and special diets are required. Mental retardation or malformations of the digestive system may cause difficulty in swallowing or digesting solid food and lead to extra expense because of the waste caused by frequent vomiting or the purchase of expensive puréed foods. The weight problems associated with poor mobility may influence families to buy more expensive high-protein food. Behavioural problems may cause parents to use food to regulate behaviour or there may be bizarre eating problems. The parents of frail children may spend more than they would normally have done on food in an attempt to improve the child's general health. Finally, the care of a very dependent child may mean that the family's food bill is higher because parents are not able to shop as efficiently or use supermarkets, relying instead on the more expensive but more convenient local shops. Eighty per cent of the children in this sample were said to have unusual eating patterns – though only 33 per cent were said actually to cost more to feed.

These subjective claims were supported by the food expenditure figures.[8] When the families with disabled children were taken as a whole their food expenditure was higher at all income levels than that of the control. As Table 6.1 indicates, the extra spent on food was not the same at all income levels, ranging from an average of £1.70 a week among the poorest to £2.19 among the richest families. When comparisons were based on the families who had actually claimed to be spending more on the disabled child's food, the difference between the samples was greater, amounting to a weekly average of £3.11 among families with net incomes of £70–£100 a week.

Table 6.1 Amount spent on food

Net weekly income (£)	Average amount spent on food each week (£)				Difference between 1 and 2 (£)
	Families with a disabled child (1)	No.	Control group (2)	No.	
Less than 70	20.86	(69)	19.16	(152)	+ 1.70
70–100	24.04	(232)	22.63	(244)	+ 1.41
100–150	26.63	(126)	24.54	(201)	+ 2.09

Obviously many gaps remain in our understanding of how a child's disablement causes extra expense on food and, even more importantly, which disabled children have food expenditure that is abnormally high. The use of average expenditure figures for large groups of families conceals the existence of a small group of families whose children's food costs are very high, either for clinical or for behavioural reasons. The following brief case-studies demonstrate some of the ways in which very high food costs can arise and how parents responded to this.

Case no. 1

This three-year-old girl was severely disabled by spina bifida and hydrocephalus. Her mother was very young, having been only eighteen when the child was born. She was an extremely conscientious mother and, even though they were very hard-pressed, said they spent a lot more on the child's food than they would normally have done. There were several reasons for this. First, they had to give her lots of drinks to help prevent bladder infections and she was unwilling to drink large quantities of water. Second, they had been advised to keep the child on a high protein diet to avoid weight problems which would hinder her mobility. Third, her mother said that because of the spina bifida her bones were more brittle and her teeth not good, so she needed extra milk and vitamins. Finally, they were extremely anxious to do the best they possibly could for the child to keep her fit and well and able to withstand infections. This in fact meant that both parents often ate badly so that the child could have protein – they had just chips when they were poor and she had fish or a piece of chicken. They estimated the *extra* cost of her food at £4 a week, though they found it difficult to do this calculation. They worried a lot when they were unable to afford what they thought of as proper food for her:

> 'I buy apples and plenty of fruit. I give her cod liver oil for her bones. Meat . . . I couldn't afford at one time to buy meat for us, but I'd always get her some kind of meat, even mince meat. . . . And if she gets too heavy she won't be able to walk, so I have to watch her weight. And the foods she needs are so expensive. Sometimes when there are bills to pay I can't afford to buy the things she needs – protein. And it preys on my mind.'

Case no. 2

This girl was twelve years old and had cystic fibrosis (CF) – basically an enzyme defect, one conseqence of which is that the child is unable to absorb fats. CF children have to follow a diet that is high in protein and vitamins and low in fats and have to eat special granules to aid in the absorption of fats. Eating the wrong foods causes pain, diarrhoea and sickness. The disease has a very poor prognosis and it is clearly important to maintain good general health as far as possible to help in withstanding chest infections. CF is also very often associated with voracious appetite. This particular child's mother very conscientiously adhered to her high-protein diet since the child was very frail. In spite of her frailty, however, when she was not ill she consumed very large quantities of food. She did not attend school, so there was plenty of opportunity for eating and her mother always had to have supplies of fruit, cheese and biscuits available for snacks. When she was ill her mother would make meals to tempt her appetite and in this way food was wasted. This woman was very reluctant to single out the disabled child by giving her special food and they ate much more meat, fish, fruit and vegetables – in and out of season – than they would normally have done on their fairly low income. (The child's father was a joiner earning £50–£60 a week at the time of the interview.) The extra costs of this child's diet were difficult to estimate and varied according to the season. However her mother estimated that the cost of her food alone was well above her lower-rate attendance allowance of £9.30 a week, the allowance being used to help with the cost of her food. Food was singled out by the parents as the most important single cost created by the condition.

In none of our analysis was any attempt made to distinguish 'necessary' from 'unnecessary' or compensatory spending on food, and this is probably impossible. For whatever reasons, around a third of the families in the sample found they were spending more on the disabled child's food. The comparative expenditure figures showed that, for those claiming they spent more, the extra cost amounted on average to £3.11 a week. The case-studies suggested that the extra ranged from under £1 a week to over £10.

Fuel

Seventy-eight per cent of the families with a disabled child said that the child's condition increased the amount of fuel they used. The commonest reason given was that the child needed extra heating – because immobility or poor circulation meant she felt the cold more, or need for attendance at night caused lighting and heating to be used during the night and early in the morning. Other reasons included heavier use of washing machines, dryers and other equipment and more use of water heaters, both for baths and for laundry for incontinent children.

The expenditure figures did not show major differences in the two samples' fuel costs. When their fuel expenditures were compared, taking the sample of families with disabled children as a whole, the poorest and middle-income families spent slightly more than the control families – 10 and 18 pence a week respectively.

The expenditure of the richest families was virtually identical (see Table 6.2). These figures suggest that disablement in a child creates a need for a small amount of extra fuel. Richer families, whose fuel expenditure is higher, can meet this need without increasing their fuel costs.

Table 6.2 Amount spent on fuel

Net weekly income (£)	Average amount spent on fuel each week (£)				Difference between 1 and 2 (£)
	Families with a disabled child (1)	No.	Control group (2)	No.	
Less than 70	5.26	(69)	5.16	(152)	+ 0.10
70–100	5.86	(233)	5.68	(244)	+ 0.18
100–150	6.11	(126)	6.10	(201)	+ 0.01

When the expenditure of the middle-income families who claimed to be spending more was scrutinized they were found to be spending an average of 31 pence a week more – £3.72 on a quarterly bill. This is not a large difference. Domestic energy costs have risen steeply since 1978 however, and the extra fuel costs of families with a disabled child may well be higher now.

The disparity between parents' own perceptions of their fuel costs and the expenditure figures is puzzling. Interviews with families showed two ways in which the amount spent on fuel can be a poor guide to families' use of fuel. First, it does not show whether families with a disabled child use their heating differently from other families or obtain very different amounts of utility or comfort from what they spend. It seems that fuel use, especially for heating, is often focused on the disabled child, whose needs are given very high priority. When these are met families cut back on fuel – sometimes to the point of discomfort – because they have other pressing needs to meet. So, for example, quite poor families would heat lavatories, bathrooms and the disabled child's bedroom or heat her bed with an electric blanket, while keeping other parts of the house unheated. A second problem is that, as with all expenditure data, we have no indication of whether the disabled child's needs *are* met, even when expenditure is relatively high. On average the differences between our two samples were not great, though they must be added to any other extra costs to be seen in perspective. It is likely, however, that there will be a small group of families whose fuel costs *are* very high. In the following brief case-studies 'extra' fuel costs and how they come about are illustrated.

Case no. 1

This eight-year-old quadriplegic boy was one of the most severely disabled children in the sample. He was almost totally helpless, incontinent, unable to communicate but not mentally handicapped. His family were extremely hard-pressed since there were three children in all and earnings from the father's job were £53 gross a week, supplemented by £10 from a part-time job by the mother, child benefit, and £21 in disability benefits. The parents said they used extra fuel for three reasons:

(a) To keep the child warm. He got about the house by rolling on the floor and therefore got very cold, so they had to heat a lot more of the house than they would otherwise have done. (He liked to roll into the hall, for example.) Since he kicked off his blankets at night his bedroom had to be heated during the night.
(b) Because of extra washing and drying from his incontinence and messy eating. They had a tumble dryer which was used often – sometimes because he was unwilling to be left alone even long enough for the clothes to be hung out.
(c) Because he needed extra baths to prevent soreness and because of incontinence.

This family installed central heating because of the child's needs. The Family Fund paid off half the cost and the remainder was borrowed from relatives to save on interest charges. This made life easier but increased their fuel bills. However they were exceptionally good managers of their money and saved every week for the bill, using the attendance allowance.

Case no. 2

This four-year-old girl suffered from Still's disease, a form of rheumatoid arthritis. Damp or cold has a very bad effect on children with this condition, causing their limbs to stiffen up. To prevent permanent stiffening it is necessary to maintain an even temperature, and this family kept their central heating, which had been installed purely because of her condition, running twenty-four hours a day, summer and winter. They also used a tumble dryer a great deal in winter and in wet weather because they could not have damp clothes around, making the atmosphere damp. Heating bills were a major problem since they were not very well off and the father had recently been unemployed for a year. During this time they had approached the supplementary benefit office for help with their gas bills but had been refused. (They had no idea what their normal fuel bills would have been and so were unable to estimate the extra cost, but said that heating was their biggest problem.)

Clothing and shoes

It is easy to understand that disability in a child may create a need for more, more expensive, or different clothing and shoes. Incontinence, hyperactivity, wear from calipers and wheelchairs, strain caused by coaxing garments on to children with awkward shapes and rigid limbs, and the wearing-out of shoes from odd gaits were among the commonest reasons given by parents in this sample for heavy wear on clothing and shoes. Previous studies have described in detail how disabilities of various sorts affect children's clothing and have suggested that a high proportion of disabled children have extra clothing needs and higher clothing costs.[9] In the present study 63 per cent of families claimed that overall expenditure on the child's clothing and shoes was higher than would be expected – allowing for some items where they spent less. More than half of these families said they spent 'a lot' more. Thirty-eight per cent of parents said that looking after the disabled child caused extra wear on their own clothes because they were soiled, caught on wheelchairs and calipers, worn out by kneeling on the floor or carrying the child or even deliberately damaged. Slightly fewer, however, said this extra wear led to their actually spending more.

The FES clothing commodity group covers both adults' and children's clothing. When the expenditure of the two samples was compared without distinguishing adults' and children's clothing no clear pattern of differences between them emerged. When expenditure on adults' and children's clothing was distinguished, however, at all income levels the families with a disabled child spent more on children's clothing, the extra ranging from an average of 8 pence a week among middle-income families to £1.82 a week among those with the highest incomes (see Table 6.3).

Table 6.3 *Amount spent on children's clothing*

Net weekly income (£)	Average amount spent on children's clothing each week (£)				Difference between 1 and 2 (£)
	Families with a disabled child (1)	No.	Control group (2)	No.	
Less than 70	1.99	(69)	1.71	(154)	+ 0.28
70–100	3.08	(233)	3.00	(244)	+ 0.08
100–150	4.73	(126)	2.91	(201)	+ 1.82

Among the families who reported that the child's condition caused extra expense on clothing the extra cost was higher – an average of 44 pence a week for families with disposable incomes of £70–£100 a week.

In both low- and middle-income families with disabled children expenditure on adults' clothing was lower than in similar control families – by 31 and 44 pence a week respectively. Parents with disabled children appear to economize on their own clothing. This may be because their budgets are under pressure, because they are less able to lead the kind of social life where clothes are important, or, more probably, for both these reasons.

Possibly even more than with other commodities, the expenditure recorded at the time of the study might not give an accurate picture of disabled children's needs for extra clothing and the way families coped with these. Interviews with parents indicated that many families with children who created heavy wear on clothing had altered the way they bought clothes. They looked for cheaper, bargain, items in sales and on market stalls and when these were found bought in bulk as far as this could be afforded. Their stocks of underwear, for example, were very large and so actual expenditure might not give a true picture of the amount bought over a year. Some children were also given a fair amount of clothing by relatives, both as presents and to help out on a regular basis. This would not be true of all the children who caused heavy wear on their clothing. It would, however, tend to depress the level of clothing expenditure for the sample so that the full cost for children not given help by relatives would be under-represented. The following brief case-studies give some idea of how disability can lead to a need for extra clothing and of families' different ways of coping with this.

Expenditure 117

Case no. 1

This thirteen-year-old girl was severely mentally handicapped and extremely hyperactive. She was also very disturbed in her behaviour and very destructive. Her parents were both professional people and had a weekly net income of over £100 a week. They said that their daughter's clothing cost a lot more than clothing for a girl of her age would normally cost, even taking into account the difference in her social life and the fact that she had less desire for fashionable clothes. The reasons for the extra cost were:

1 General roughness and clumsiness in dressing and undressing and in playing. She fights a lot at school and often comes home with torn clothes.
2 Messiness and spells of incontinence.
3 Needing bigger clothes. She is very large and takes a large adult's size in clothing.
4 Wanton destructiveness. She cuts clothes up deliberately or tears them. (She also cuts them by mistake as when during the interview she was cutting out a paper pattern and cut her dress with it.)

This extra wear applied to most of her clothing. Though her parents said they did not spend extra money in attempting to minimize her handicap or compensate her, neither were they willing, as people had suggested, to buy very cheap clothes because they would only be destroyed.

Case no. 2

This fourteen-year-old girl had spina bifida. She was paralysed below the waist, got around by wheelchair and had a urinary diversion. It might have been expected that incontinence and rubbing by her wheelchair would lead to extra spending on clothes, while some compensatory spending on clothes would have been very understandable for a girl of her age. Her mother was, however, determined to treat her as normally as possible. They were also very hard-pressed financially since her father was an unskilled labourer. Her parents said in the interview that they spent nothing extra at all on the child's clothes. Though she did wear out the sleeves of her cardigans and jumpers, lots of clothes were handed on to her by friends and her grandmother also gave her clothes. Since she was big and an odd shape she had clothes made by her grandmother which worked out cheaper. She did not go out as normally a girl of her age would to parties and discos, and so did not need expensive fashionable clothes. She did wear out anoraks with the wheelchair, but since she could not wear coats, which were more expensive, this cancelled out the extra expense. Her mother was adamant, too, that she did not believe in compensatory spending.

> 'I know it sounds awful, but it's not my fault. It nearly broke my heart when she was born, but I went into it and I know it wasn't my fault. I try to make it up to her – she's got a good home and parents that love her – but I don't spoil her . . . I don't buy things for her, part because I can't afford it and part because I don't want to make her mean and peevish.'

This woman said their only extra clothing expense was probably for the disabled child's sister, who had to have new things instead of having them handed down as would normally have happened.

Transport

The importance of transport for families with a disabled child is obvious and well documented.[10] The practical difficulties of moving around with children in wheelchairs or with gross behavioural problems, the danger of social isolation and the need to maintain contact with schools, hospitals and other agencies all make access to convenient and flexible forms of transport desirable. Being without such transport can cause isolation and stress.

Given the importance of transport to families with disabled children one might expect their transport expenditure to be higher than that of the control families. Car ownership and expenditure on petrol might be a necessity of life for these families rather than a luxury. However we know that their incomes are lower, and that even when their cash incomes are the same as other families' they are poorer in real terms because the child's condition creates extra needs for items such as food and fuel. Since transport *can* be economized on without risking health it would not be surprising, therefore, to find some economizing among the poorest families with disabled children. Fewer of these families might run cars, for example, or those who owned cars might ration their use fairly stringently. Moreover, some children might be so severely disabled that, even with access to cars, getting about outside is very difficult.

The transport expenditure of this sample of families with a disabled child was strongly influenced by their incomes. In general they spent substantially more than similar FES families and the extra they spent increased with income. Middle-income families with a disabled child spent on average £2.10 a week more than similar FES families (see Table 6.4). Among high-income families, whose basic transport expenditure was in any case higher, the *extra* cost of transport rose to an average of £5.47 a week more. Clearly there is great potential for high transport expenditure when a child is disabled.

As Table 6.4 shows, the poorest families in both samples spent considerably less on transport than families in the higher income ranges. Strikingly, however, the poorest families with a disabled child also spent less on transport than their FES counterparts – an average of 51 pence a week. There is no reason to believe that the need for transport of poor families with disabled children is less than that of families with more money. Their lower transport expenditure can only be an indication of unmet need.

Table 6.4 Amount spent on transport

Net weekly income (£)	Average amount spent on transport each week (£)				Difference between 1 and 2 (£)
	Families with a disabled child (1)	No.	Control group (2)	No.	
Less than 70	6.60	(69)	7.11	(152)	− 0.51
70–100	12.28	(233)	10.17	(244)	+ 2.11
100–150	19.25	(126)	13.78	(201)	+ 5.47

Isolating the expenditure of the families who claimed to be spending more on transport considerably widened the gap between the FES control and this sample of families with disabled children. For families with disposable incomes of £70–£100 a week the difference in the average weekly expenditure of the families who said the child's condition caused them to spend more on transport and that of the control families was £3.42 a week.

Transport expenditure was strongly influenced by whether families were receiving mobility allowances. Among middle-income families those with mobility allowances were spending an average of £5.33 a week more on transport than those without and £6.86 a week more than the control. However, even when they did not have mobility allowances, middle-income families with disabled children spent more than the control families on transport, the difference in their average weekly transport expenditure being £1.53.

The foregoing expenditure figures, which relate to all types of transport expenditure, are dominated by expenditure on the purchase and maintenance of cars. Expenditure on petrol is probably a more sensitive indicator of the disabled child's day-to-day transport costs. At all income levels the families with disabled children spent more on petrol than the control families, the difference in expenditure increasing with income and ranging from an average of 25 pence a week among the poorest families to £1.61 among the richest. The 'extra cost' of the families who claimed that the child's condition caused them to spend more on petrol (56 per cent of the sample) was higher – an average of £3.23 a week among middle-income families.

Receipt of mobility allowance did not have a striking impact on petrol expenditure. The petrol expenditures of families with and without mobility allowance were fairly similar, both being higher than the petrol expenditure of the control. This suggests that mobility allowances were being used by the families in this sample to purchase cars, or more suitable cars, rather than for extra or longer journeys with the child. It also suggests, if petrol expenditure is a reliable indicator of need, that the current mobility allowance criteria do not accurately identify the families who need help with their transport costs. A sizeable group of families not receiving mobility allowances spent almost as much on petrol as those who did receive them. Presumably they were driving older, and possibly less suitable, vehicles. The following case-studies give some idea of the way children's disabilities affected the transport costs of families who did and did not receive mobility allowances.

Case no. 1

This severely disabled four-year-old boy had a severe congenital heart defect and had also been born with a cleft palate and harelip. At the time of the interview he was awaiting major heart surgery but was not yet old enough or well enough for surgery. He was unable to walk more than a hundred yards without tiring and suffered from heart failure sometimes – especially in windy weather. He had one other brother, his father was a fairly low-paid unskilled labourer and the family could not afford to run a car. They lived five miles away from the nearest town, in a village, and saw transport and isolation, particularly for the mother, as their main problem. They were unable to use public transport, both because the child's still open cleft palate and lung weakness made him vulnerable to infections and because he had to be pushed in a wheelchair and carried while on the bus if there was no seat. His heart failure and proneness to temper tantrums added to the difficulties of using public transport. This meant that for the child to get out at all they had to use taxis and in an average week reckoned to spend £2 to get him to playgroup and back once and £2 to go once to the nearest town. The child was very demanding and the mother very stressed, especially in a week when they could not afford a taxi to get out. At the time of the interview they were unable to spend much on taxis because they had just decided to buy their local authority house and this had meant an increase of £16 a week in their housing costs. By the time this child was old enough to qualify for a mobility allowance it is possible that he would no longer need it, having had his heart operation. The family's transport costs, however, started to be a problem soon after his birth, they thought, and were a big problem after he was about two.

Case no. 2

This child was thirteen, quadriplegic, spastic and very dependent. He did not attend school because there was no suitable place for him – he was of normal intelligence but so dependent that he needed special care and the only local special-care unit was for children who were severely mentally handicapped. He was, and for eight years had been, totally unable to use public transport. His family was not at all well off since his father was a self-employed accountant, earning £56 a week net and working from home, having been made redundant two years previously. In spite of this they ran two cars. One was needed so that the father could visit clients. The second was to prevent the mother from being totally isolated. Since the child was at home all the time she would not have been able to go out without a car. They had a Mini, which they used for driving around town, and a larger four-door estate car for use when they were travelling any distance and had to take wheelchair, special food, changes of clothes and nappies, drinks and so on. The cost of running two cars on their present income was a strain but was something they felt they could not manage without. They tried to use the cars as moderately as possible but made strenuous efforts to help the child lead as full a life as possible, taking him for example to folk and transport museums, farms, air-shows, country houses and so on. The child had no speech and could communicate with his parents but not easily with strangers and they clearly felt very responsible for compensating as far as possible for his lack of companionship with other children. The mobility allowance helped with, but obviously did not cover, their transport costs, and there were clear signs of economies on other things such as heating, television, furniture and clothes for both parents.

Up to this point we have been considering expenditure which can be directly linked with the disabled child. For the next two commodities considered – alcohol and tobacco – such a direct link cannot be made. Expenditure on alcohol and tobacco can, nevertheless, be linked to the presence of severe disablement in a child, albeit less directly. Parents' ability to spend on both may be affected by the need to provide for the disabled child's special needs, while restrictions on their social lives may lead to involuntary savings on, for example, drinks in clubs and pubs. It is equally possible, however, that the physical and emotional stresses of caring for a very dependent child may cause parents to smoke and drink more than they would normally have done.

Alcohol

At all income levels families with a disabled child spent less on alcohol than the FES control, the difference varying from an average of 47 pence a week among the richest families to 87 pence among those with the lowest incomes (see Table 6.5). This finding was not unexpected. When interviewed in depth families frequently mentioned their inability to go out together socially as a major source of discontent. In most cases this was due to difficulties in finding suitable care for the disabled child. However lack of money was also given as a reason why men in particular were said not to go out as often as they would have done to pubs or clubs or spent less when they did go out.

Table 6.5 Amount spent on alcohol

Net weekly income (£)	Average amount spent on alcohol each week (£)				
	Families with a disabled child (1)	No.	Control group (2)	No.	Difference between 1 and 2 (£)
Less than 70	2.13	(69)	3.00	(152)	− 0.87
70–100	2.54	(233)	3.25	(244)	− 0.71
100–150	2.78	(126)	3.25	(201)	− 0.47

Tobacco

At all income levels the families with a disabled child spent more on tobacco than similar families in the control, the extra ranging from 56 pence a week among middle incomes families to £1.28 a week among those with the lowest incomes (see Table 6.6). This picture of higher tobacco expenditure among the families with disabled children remained when tobacco expenditure was analysed for non-manual and manual workers separately. The recent reduction in smoking among higher income groups appears not to have occurred to the same extent among families with a disabled child. It may be that high tobacco expenditure reflects the stress associated with caring for a disabled child and also the much lower proportion of women going out to work. Women who are at home all day without company have more opportunity for smoking and are also more likely to experience stress.

Table 6.6 Amount spent on tobacco

Net weekly income (£)	Average amount spent on tobacco each week (£)				
	Families with a disabled child (1)	No.	Control group (2)	No.	Difference between 1 and 2 (£)
Less than 70	4.29	(69)	3.01	(152)	+ 1.28
70–100	3.14	(233)	2.58	(244)	+ 0.56
100–150	3.15	(126)	2.52	(201)	+ 0.63

Expenditure on the remaining FES commodity groups is less easy to link directly to the presence of disablement in a child. In the case of durable household goods the infrequency of purchases means that differences between the samples over time may be masked. For services, other and miscellaneous goods, which are large and heterogeneous groupings, average expenditure figures may conceal the effect of the child's condition: extra expenditure needed on one item may be found by economizing on others and no overall difference in expenditure appear. The services commodity group, for example, includes telephone costs, which are likely to be higher among families with a disabled child. It also includes the cost of cinema and theatre tickets, hairdressing and other 'luxuries' on which they may economize. For this reason from time to time we compare expenditure on particular items claimed by families to cost more because of the child's condition.

Durable household goods

This commodity group includes both furniture and other household furnishings and consumer durables like refrigerators, washing machines and television sets. Previous research has consistently found large numbers of parents claiming that the child's condition affected their expenditure on such items – either by causing them to be bought at all or by the need to replace them more frequently than would normally be expected.[11] Of the families in this sample 36 per cent said that the child's equipment, notably wheelchairs, caused damage to fittings and carpets. Fifty-six per cent said that various aspects of the condition itself – incontinence, vomiting, destructiveness – caused damage to furniture and carpets. Acquiring items such as telephones, washing machines, freezers and other consumer durables was frequently related to the child's condition.

Table 6.7 Amount spent on durable household goods

Net weekly income (£)	Average amount spent on durable household goods each week (£)				Difference between 1 and 2 (£)
	Families with a disabled child (1)	No.	Control group (2)	No.	
Less than 70	6.52	(69)	3.54	(152)	+ 2.98
70–100	5.92	(233)	5.08	(144)	+ 0.84
100–150	6.59	(126)	6.41	(201)	+ 0.18

As Table 6.7 shows, expenditure on durable household goods supports the claim that families with disabled children spend more on these goods. The much higher amount spent by the poorest families (an average of £2.98 a week) and the way the 'extra cost' declines as incomes rise suggests that, as families themselves reported, the child's condition forced them to acquire assets they could not really afford. At higher incomes families would be buying such items in any case.

Services

As already noted, this commodity group covers both services where the families with disabled children might be expected to spend more and some where they might be expected to economize. On balance it would appear that economy prevailed (see Table 6.8). At all income levels the families with a disabled child spent less than similar control families, the amount less ranging from 20 pence a week among middle-income families to 52 pence a week among those with the lowest incomes. However, there were particular services on which the families with disabled children spent more than their FES counterparts. Their telephone bills, for example, were an average of £3.60 a quarter higher than those of the control families, supporting the claims of parents that they made heavier use of their telephones to keep in touch with services and to reduce isolation. Somewhat unexpectedly, the families with a disabled child also spent more on entertainment outside the home than similar control families, the amount extra ranging from 18 pence a week among poor families to £1.13 among those with the highest incomes. Our interviews with parents suggested that this higher expenditure was on the children in the family, rather than on adults: parents reported spending more than they would

Table 6.8 Amount spent on services

Net weekly income (£)	Average amount spent on services each week (£)				
	Families with a disabled child (1)	No.	Control group (2)	No.	Difference between 1 and 2 (£)
Less than 70	3.90	(69)	4.42	(152)	− 0.52
70–100	6.02	(233)	5.82	(244)	+ 0.20
100–150	8.44	(126)	8.91	(201)	− 0.47

normally have done on entertainment of various sorts to improve the disabled child's quality of life, or to compensate other children for lack of parental attention.

Housing costs

Table 6.9 shows the two samples' housing costs – i.e. rent, rates and mortgage costs, plus insurance on the structure of the house and routine repairs and maintenance. As this table shows, low-and middle-income families with a disabled child spent less than similar families in the control while those in the highest income group spent slightly more.

Table 6.9 Amount spent on housing

Net weekly income (£)	Average amount spent on housing each week (£)				Difference between 1 and 2 (£)
	Families with a disabled child (1)	No.	Control group (2)	No.	
Less than 70	7.69	(69)	8.25	(152)	– 0.56
70–100	11.34	(233)	12.80	(244)	– 1.46
100–150	18.27	(126)	17.99	(201)	+ 0.28

It should be stressed that these figures provide only a crude, and possibly misleading measure of the extent to which a child's disablement may affect a family's housing costs.[12] The costs of adapting houses are not included here. Moreover in the longer term the child's condition may affect the family's housing tenure. Like previous studies of disabled children,[13] the present study found a significantly lower proportion of both non-manual and manual families with a disabled child in owner-occupied housing. In the short term this is likely to mean that the housing costs of families with disabled children are lower. This has to be weighed against longer-term financial effects, particularly the loss of capital appreciation from owner-occupation. Our interviews revealed that some families with disabled children regarded being unable to buy a house as one of the longer-term effects of the child's disablement on their financial position and very much regretted this. Clearly, such longer-term effects will not adequately be reflected by cross-sectional data on housing costs. The disabled child's effect on families' housing is discussed further below with other less regular costs (pp. 132–4).

Other and miscellaneous goods

This residual expenditure category covers a wide range of items some of which, such as toilet goods and proprietary medicines, might well be affected by disablement. However most of the other items in this category bear no obvious relation to disablement – jewellery and fancy goods, plants and seeds and photographic goods for example.[14]

Only among the poorest families did any marked difference in expenditure emerge at the broad commodity group level, the families with disabled children spending on average £1.42 a week more than similar control families. The expenditure of families in the other income ranges was virtually identical (see Table 6.10). Expenditure figures for particular items did support parents' claims that the child's condition caused extra expense, though the extra amount involved was small: an average, among middle-income families, of 26 pence a week extra on cleaning materials, 10 pence on proprietary medicines and 30 pence on toys and other recreational materials.

Table 6.10 Amount spent on other and miscellaneous goods

Net weekly income (£)	Average amount spent on other and miscellaneous goods each week (£)				Difference between 1 and 2 (£)
	Families with a disabled child (1)	No.	Control group (2)	No.	
Less than 70	5.73	(69)	4.31	(152)	+ 1.42
70–100	6.64	(233)	6.58	(244)	+ 0.06
100–150	8.24	(126)	8.36	(201)	− 0.12

The foregoing analysis has explored the disabled child's effect on expenditure by comparing the average weekly expenditure of families in three broad income ranges. As a method of analysing expenditure patterns this is fairly crude. However, when multiple regression analysis was used to overcome some of its limitations the picture that emerged was substantially unaltered.[15] Again, there was clear evidence that most of the families with disabled children had extra costs. Interestingly, however, this analysis revealed that on a number of commodities where most families with disabled children spent more than the control, the poorest families with disabled children were spending less. This was true of food, transport and children's clothing. This suggests that for the poorest families the scope for meeting the disabled child's special needs is very limited. They can only be met, if at all, by stringent economies. The quality of life of such families and of the disabled children in them must be a cause for concern.

Adding up the costs

The figures presented above show that severe disablement in a child caused most families in this sample to spend more than their FES counterparts on a number of individual items. They tell us nothing, however, about the overall impact on families' budgets – how much extra was spent each week in meeting the child's special needs. In this section, therefore, we look at this overall cost. As will become clear, the overall cost to families can be defined and measured in a number of ways, with different results. A range of estimates based on different assumptions is therefore presented. These estimates are subject to important qualifications – most importantly that they do not reflect the variations in cost that undoubtedly exist because disabled children vary greatly in their needs. The figures that follow should therefore be regarded as a rough guide to the extra cost of disablement in a child, not as a precise measure of this cost.

In investigating the overall cost of the child's disablement families were again grouped into three broad income ranges. Here, to simplify what would otherwise be a very complicated picture, detailed figures are presented only for families in the middle-income range. There are, in any case, strong reasons for focusing on this group of families. It is the largest group – containing 54 per cent of the families with a disabled child and 41 per cent of the control. Information on expenditure differences is more reliable, therefore, than for the other groups. Middle-income families are also a useful reference group for policy purposes, illustrating the costs of a child's disablement for 'typical' families rather than those whose spending is constrained by poverty or who can spend freely because they are rich.[16]

The cost of disablement in a child will depend on the income level at which comparisons with other families are made. It will also depend on how the cost to families is defined. A number of approaches is possible. We can, for example, compare the total amount of money families spend each week, assuming that any surplus spending by the families with a disabled child represents the 'extra cost' of disablement. An alternative approach is to add up any extra spent on particular items. Both these methods are used below.

It could be argued that account should also be taken of the way disablement can alter the way money is allocated within families and the utility families obtain from what they buy. As we have seen, families spending much the same as their FES counterparts on heating or toilet requisites did not always benefit to the same extent because these items were used mainly for the disabled child. Quantifying such differences in use is extremely difficult, however, and has not been attempted here.

Table 6.11 shows the two groups' average weekly expenditures on the main FES commodity groups. As these figures show, the total expenditure of the families with disabled children was higher, on average, than that of the control families. On the assumption that families met the child's special needs simply by spending more of their incomes each week the extra cost of the child's

Table 6.11 Average weekly expenditure on all commodities by families with disposable incomes of £70–£100 a week

Commodity	Families with a disabled child (1) £	No.	Control group (2) £	No.	Difference (1–2)
Food	24.04	233	22.63	244	+ 1.41
Fuel	5.86		5.68		+ 0.18
Transport and vehicles	12.27		10.17		+ 2.10
Tobacco	3.14		2.58		+ 0.56
Durable household goods	5.92		5.08		+ 0.84
Services	6.02		5.82		+ 0.20
Other & miscellaneous goods	6.64		6.58		+ 0.06
Clothing	6.39		6.75		– 0.36
- children's	3.08		3.00		+ 0.08
- adults'	3.31		3.75		– 0.44
Alcohol	2.54		3.25		– 0.71
Housing	11.34		12.80		– 1.46
Total expenditure	84.16		81.34		+ 2.82

	1978 prices	1984 prices
Difference in total expenditure	£2.82	£5.10
Extra spent on FES commodity groups	£5.43	£9.83

disablement in 1978, for middle-income families, was £2.82 a week – £5.07 at 1984 prices.[17]

A closer reading of Table 6.11 suggests that the disabled child's needs are met, not only by spending more of the family's income, but also by altering the way money is spent: spending more on things that are needed by the child and economizing on others. On this view the extra cost of the child's disablement can more accurately be estimated by adding up the extra spent by the families with disabled children on those commodities where they spent more than the control group. This gives a total extra cost, in 1978 of £5.43 – just under £10 at 1984 prices.

This total does not take into account the extra spending we have identified on individual items within the main commodity groups, such as children's clothing, telephone calls and entertainment outside the home. Including such items would bring the total extra cost of this group of families with disabled children to at least £6.50 a week in 1978 – around £12 at 1984 prices.

The crudity of this approach to measuring the overall cost of the child's disablement must be acknowledged. Reservations must be expressed, for example, about the weight that can be attached to average extra cost figures when so little is known about variations in extra spending. Disabled children vary greatly in their needs. Information from parents suggested that both the numbers spending extra on particular items and the amount spent varied greatly. FES expenditure data are not, unfortunately, suitable for analysis at the level of individuals or very small groups,[18] hence such variations in extra cost cannot be identified. The overall extra cost figures presented above can therefore not be taken as the amount spent by *most* families in this income range. Some may spend much more, some much less – though investigation of families' typical 'package' of extra costs suggested that very few families had no, or very little, extra expense.[19]

Moreover even the highest estimate quoted above is likely to understate the true impact of the child's disablement. Since FES expenditure data do not allow spending on particular individuals to be identified, the extent to which the disabled child's needs are met at the expense of other family members is hidden. Parents in this study spoke of eating poorer food so that the disabled child could eat well; economizing on heating so that the child's bedroom could be kept warm; using the telephone or car mainly for the disabled child.

Expenditure 131

Changes in the purposes for which items are bought are also hidden. The toiletries bought by the control families, for example, will usually serve the whole family and will often contain an element of luxury spending. Those bought by families with disabled children are more likely to be utilitarian items needed in the management of incontinence. As already noted, these subtler effects on expenditure patterns and in the utility derived from what is bought cannot be captured from FES data – though our interviews with parents suggested that they were very common.

The effect of income on extra costs

The figures quoted so far refer to families in the middle-income range. For those in the lowest and highest income ranges a similar pattern emerged – though the total amount of extra money spent varied considerably with income. Table 6.12 summarizes the disabled child's effect on expenditure for families in all three income ranges.

In each income range the families with disabled children spent more, in total, each week than the control families. However the extra was greater among the richest and poorest families than for those in the middle-income range. Calculating the overall cost from expenditure on individual items produced a similar picture of higher extra costs among the richest and poorest families.

It may seem strange that the extra cost of bringing up a disabled child should be higher for the poorest families than for those who are slightly better off. The explanation is probably that providing for the child's special needs forces the poorest families to live beyond their means. These special needs are much less likely to be met within the normal budgets of families with very low incomes. They spend much more than they would normally do on things like consumer durables, for example, and much more than control families with similar incomes. Middle-income families are more likely to own cars and other consumer durables already. Hence the *extra* spent as a result of the child's condition is smaller – though the total amount spent on her will be higher than in poorer families.

It might have been expected, then, that among the richest families the extra cost of the child's disablement would be even smaller. Table 6.12 shows that this was not so; it was substantially higher than that of families with lower incomes. However, the families in the middle-income range were spending all – and in some cases more than – their incomes.[20] Clearly, as more money becomes available it continues to be directed disproportionately to the disabled child. There appears to be no income point at which the child's special needs are met within the family's normal budget. The potential for using money to improve the child's, or the family's, quality of life seems virtually infinite.

Table 6.12 Total extra cost of disablement at different income levels (£ p.w.)

Disposable income	Difference in total expenditure		Extra on FES Commodity groups	
	1978 prices	1984 prices	1978 prices	1984 prices
Less than 70	4.99	9.00	7.76	14.05
70–100	2.82	5.10	5.43	9.83
100–150	9.77	17.68	10.58	19.15

The finding that income so strongly influences the cost of disablement in a child has interesting implications for policy and for the basis on which increased financial help might be given to families. These questions are discussed in the concluding chapter of this book. For the moment it is sufficient to note that at all income levels disablement in a child substantially altered families' regular spending patterns. Though important questions remain about variations in the extra cost the comparative expenditure data from this study demonstrate clearly that severe disablement adds substantially to the normal costs of child-raising.

Less regular expenditure

As was noted earlier, comparative expenditure data based on short time periods may not accurately reflect the special expenses that can arise from time to time. Parents were questioned directly about four such possible types of expense: housing, special equipment, consumer durables and contacts with hospitals. Where appropriate they were asked how much they had spent on these items in the preceding two years. In all four areas many families had incurred expense, though the number of families and the amounts spent varied considerably.[21]

Housing

Finding or creating suitable housing had presented problems for the majority of families. It had been a major and expensive problem for a smaller group – predominantly those who were buying their houses and whose child was very severely disabled – typically wheelchair-bound and incontinent. Forty-six per cent of the sample had moved to their present housing solely on the disabled child's account; 55 per cent had adapted houses to make it easier to care for the child or give her more independence. The average amount spent on adaptations by parents themselves in the previous two years was £364. However 15 families had spent more than £1,000, while the highest amount spent was £4,000.

Special equipment

Special equipment was apparently easier to obtain from the statutory authorities than housing adaptations. Though the majority of the children in the study relied on such equipment very few had paid for it themselves. Ninety-eight per cent of the sample had spent something on aids, equipment or special furniture in the preceding two years. However the amounts spent were relatively small: an average of £71 on mobility aids; £26 on aids to communication; £5 on aids to personal independence and £37 on special furniture. However when the cost of housing adaptations was included the average amount spent in the preceding two years was £184.

Consumer durables

Parents frequently related their purchase of items such as cars, washing machines and telephones to the child's disablement. Some were needed in the everyday management of the condition: freezers to store special foods, for example, or automatic washing machines where children were incontinent. Others, such as dishwashers, were used as a way of buying time for parents under pressure. Finally, items such as stereo equipment and colour television had often been bought to improve the quality of life of the disabled child and other members of the family – particularly when social life outside the home was restricted.

Consumer durables and furnishings were also said to need

replacing more frequently – cars and washing machines because of heavy use; furniture and carpets because they were damaged by wheelchairs, soiled by incontinence or destroyed by children whose behaviour was disturbed. Unlike special equipment consumer durables were usually paid for by families themselves, with the exception of washing machines and tumble dryers, where the Family Fund was a frequent source of supply.

Some families said they had bought items they would not normally have bought at all. More frequently it was the timing of the purchase that was said to be different. Things were bought sooner than would normally have been expected and before they could strictly be afforded. Replacing more expensive items loomed as a major problem, especially when, as not infrequently happened, they wore out before they had been completely paid for.

Surprisingly, comparison with the control families' ownership of five common consumer durables – cars, refrigerators, central heating, telephones and washing machines – showed that ownership of some of these items was *less* common among the families with disabled children. This was particularly true of the poorest families.

At all income levels the families with disabled children were less likely to have central heating than the control families. The poorest families with disabled children were also less likely to have cars and refrigerators. Only in the case of washing machines and telephones was ownership higher among the families with disabled children at all income levels. Their higher ownership of washing machines reflects Family Fund policy of supplying these to families whose disabled children are incontinent. The cost of telephones, on the other hand, would usually be met by families themselves. Clearly, when a child is disabled telephones are regarded more as a necessity than as a luxury.

It is not surprising that poorer families with disabled children are less likely than families with similar incomes to own expensive consumer durables. The child's higher everyday costs must make these difficult to afford. It is regrettable, however, given the demands that severely disabled children can make on their parents' time and energy, that poorer families are less likely to own the labour-saving equipment owned both by more prosperous families with disabled children and by control families with similar incomes.

Hospital costs
Hospitals loom large in the lives of many disabled children, both for out-patient appointments and when they are admitted for treatment. It is a cardinal principle of the National Health Service that medical care is free. However using health services can involve considerable costs where children are concerned: apart from the more obvious costs of getting to hospitals and loss of earnings by parents escorting or visiting them, a number of less obvious costs can arise. Paying for other young children to be looked after while parents are at hospital is one example.

Parents in this study were asked about costs arising both from out-patient visits and from admissions. The great majority – 95 per cent – bore the cost of travel to out-patient appointments themselves, travelling by car or public transport. Earnings were frequently lost by one or both parents on these occasions and money had often to be spent on meals. In general these costs could be absorbed, though problems could arise when visits were very frequent. Greater problems arose when children had to go regularly to specialist hospitals a long way from their homes. This involved expensive fares for the child and often both parents, the cost of meals and the loss of a day's wages. For poorer families finding the money could be difficult. The parents of a child with a rare skin complaint, for example, who had to travel frequently from their home in a small Cheshire village to Great Ormond Street Hospital in London, found these visits a great financial strain, since the man was a low-paid agricultural worker.

In general, however, though causing some financial strain, out-patient appointments did not cause severe financial stress. This was not true of going into hospital.

Whatever the reason for the child's admission parents were likely to encounter expenses – for new pyjamas and presents for the child, for their own fares to hospital and from earnings lost in visiting. Almost half of the children in the sample had been admitted to hospital in the previous year. More than 80 per cent of them had been visited at least once a day by parents; only 8 per cent had received any help with visiting costs.

The greatest financial disruption occurred when children were very ill and the outcome was uncertain or when major or painful treatment was required. Children born with major impairments requiring surgery, those undergoing treatment for cancers or renal failure, and those requiring complicated urinary tract operations were all likely to involve families in financial as well as emotional stress. Where hospitals were far away or difficult to reach by public transport, the hospital stay was prolonged, and there were other young children in the family, the difficulties increased. These difficulties were caused not only by parental earnings loss and the costs of visiting children but also by the difficulty of adhering to normal budgeting patterns. Parents tended to live from hand to mouth, subordinating everything to the disabled child's needs and borrowing money when it was needed. The following case-study illustrates the severe financial stress that can be associated with admission to hospital.

This thirteen-year-old boy experienced renal failure when he was nine. Between then and being eleven and a half he spent much of his time in hospital. The first eight months of his illness were spent entirely in hospital on dialysis, with little hope being given of his survival. After two and a half years he had a kidney transplant which lasted for thirteen months and was then rejected. After another period of hospitalization and dialysis he received another kidney transplant which up to the time of the study had been successful.

The periods spent, over four years, in hospital were too numerous for the family to be able to itemize. In the first year, however, altogether ten months were spent in three hospitals, the hospital where most time was spent being 36 miles away. The lengths of time in hospital varied but could last up to four months. When he was at home he had frequently to be rushed back into hospital if he showed signs of illness.

The emotional strain on this family, in the first two years of their son's illness particularly, was enormous. The financial strain was also immense. They were a fairly hard-pressed family with no savings and two other small children. The man was an unskilled labourer. In the first two years of the boy's illness the family received no help from any statutory source though they were paying very high transport costs, buying toys and other things to keep the sick child amused and keep his spirits up, and paying for child-minding for the other children. It was not till the boy had been ill for two years, the father's health was giving way and they had accumulated enormous debts to relatives that they finally began looking for financial help from sources outside relatives and friends. The first approach they made at that point was to the local supplementary benefit office who were unable to help because the man was in full-time work. The man's employers, however, stepped in, giving him a lighter job and the use of the firm's van for hospital visits. The parents also heard of the attendance allowance at this point and were awarded the higher rate. In the period after that, though things were still very difficult, they were less desperate than in the early stages of the boy's illness.

The boy's mother described, graphically, how their entire budgeting strategy broke down under the strains of continual uncertainty about their son's survival and totally unpredictable demands for money. Their first priority was always to get to hospital; money itself was of secondary importance:

'It was all one big mess. We were in a complete mess. Taking from Peter to pay Paul. And we couldn't ever sit down to work out our money because we already owed what we'd coming in, from the week before. And we couldn't see a way out of the mess ahead, at all. . . . Money wasn't a problem before. We managed to live from week to week and pay our bills. We were no more in debt than anyone else. I mean everybody's got their club people, haven't they? We always paid them without having to borrow the money. We got into trouble when John was ill because we just hadn't the money behind us, to cope. . . . We used to spend so much time at the hospital, the girl next door but one – my littlest one used to call her "mum". He didn't know his own mother. And you couldn't expect people to sit, day in, day out, night in, night out watching children without giving them anything at all. . . . We used to give her what we could afford – whatever we had in our pockets – fifty pence, twenty pence. We'd pay her about a pound or thirty bob a week. If we had it we'd give her it, if we hadn't we'd make it up another week. It wasn't a lot, but when it's all expense on expense, added up, you can't cope. . . . The time he was ill, we couldn't get no money from anywhere, you see. To be quite honest, we hadn't the money to spend on food. We used to be down to one meal a day when John was ill. Not so much that we hadn't got time to eat, or even feel like it. It was as much as we could afford. Don't misunderstand me. John got his, and the children. But *we've* gone without many and many a meal. We've been up the hospital and had a bag of crisps. Gone all day on a bag of crisps and a cup of coffee. We used to get a cup of coffee out of the machine and have a bag of crisps. When we got fed up with the crisps we'd have a little packet of biscuits. Because, you see, we had to watch the money, with the travelling. . . . We were *desperately* in financial difficulties. We were borrowing left, right and centre. I mean, I've only just finished paying my auntie back, and it's only going to work myself that's made us able to pay her back hundreds of pounds that we borrowed just to be able to go and see John. I can honestly say, of all the times he's been in hospital, we've never, never missed a day. And it's not just the petrol for the car, it's tax and insurance and repairs because you never know when you'll need that car. We've practically borrowed his wages, often, before he got paid – just to live, and paid them back on Friday and then had to borrow it again on Sunday and Monday. I just last week paid off the last of our rent arrears. . . . We borrowed pounds and pounds. We've just, and when I say just I mean *just* – last week actually, come up to date with our payments. After all that time.'

Renal failure is, fortunately, rare. However commoner conditions can also cause financial stress when children are admitted to hospital. A nine-year-old boy with spina bifida, for example, had been admitted six times for surgery. A year previously he had been admitted for three weeks for surgery on his urinary tract. He was an only child and both his parents were employed. Since he was having a major operation his father took two weeks off work without pay and a week of his annual holiday so that he could visit each day. His wife lost three weeks' pay. Their combined earnings loss amounted, in 1977, to £250, while their other costs amounted, they estimated, to £150:

'At that time [i.e. 1977] we reckoned it cost us £150 . . . for petrol, food, new pyjamas and bits of presents for David. And you've got to be decent yourself, you know. New tights and that. . . . And then you're snacking down there in the café. You rush out in the morning without a proper breakfast and by eleven o'clock you're starving so you go down for a cup of tea and a bun or something. And there's your lunch. And then when you get home at night you're exhausted, so you buy fish and chips for supper or something, and that's dearer. At the time it's funny how you manage. Where you find the money from. You think, "Well how are we going to cope?" But you do.

But it's months and months before you recover. . . . You just can't ever seem to get into a routine with your money. I'm still not straight from the last time. We've never yet been able to put money away for bills.'

Parents are increasingly encouraged to spent time with their children when they are in hospital. The financial implications of doing so can be considerable, particularly for the parents of disabled children whose budgets are already tight and who have little to fall back on. There is no adequate statutory source of financial help with hospital costs. Indeed, when children have been in hospital more than four weeks their entitlement to attendance allowance stops – even though mothers in particular spend a large part of each day with the child. The case for improving financial support to families whose children are in hospital, rather than cutting existing support, is very strong.

Summary

In this, as in other studies, parents of disabled children reported that the child's condition created extra costs. This claim was tested in relation to everyday living costs, larger items bought less frequently and the episodic costs associated with hospital treatment. In all three areas it was clear that the child's disablement had led to extra expense and had substantially altered families' expenditure patterns.

An important finding to emerge from this analysis was that the 'extra cost' of severe disablement in a child was not a fixed amount but varied in a complicated way with family income. This means that it is not possible to produce one summary figure for the child's costs which could, for example, be used to determine the appropriate level for an extra costs allowance. The extra cost of disablement depends on the income point at which comparisons are made. However for the middle-income families in this study nothing less than £12 a week (at 1984 costs) would have had a significant impact on their regular extra costs. If account were taken of the less regular costs arising from the need for housing adaptations, the purchase and replacement of consumer durables and hospital costs the figure would be much higher.

In the following chapter we look briefly at how these families with disabled children adapted to and coped with the financial constraints imposed by the child's condition, how they perceived the effect on their living standards and what help they thought was appropriate.

7 The overall effect – ways of coping and expectations of help

In this chapter we look at the overall effect of the child's disablement on families' living standards and how they responded to this. This is done, not by combining figures on income losses and extra expense to produce an overall 'cost' in money terms but by documenting the effect as parents themselves saw it.

Strategies for coping

For some families the disabled child's effect on their finances or living standards is minimal. Where the family's income is reasonable, the child's condition moderate and stable, and services good, no effect may be noticed. Any financial loss will be covered by attendance and mobility allowances: where families are receiving both higher-rate attendance and mobility allowances and there have been no major capital costs, the impact is less likely to be very great. It will be even less when there is no substantial effect on parental earnings.

These conditions were met for a very small minority of families in this study. In this chapter, therefore, we look mainly at those who do experience some financial effect. How did these families manage?

The first, and most obvious, point to be made is that like most people faced with particular tasks or problems families with disabled children respond to the financial 'problem' posed by disablement by developing coping strategies. Our analysis of employment patterns indicated, for example, that some men increased their hours of work in response to their wives' inability to go out to work, while some women limited demands on their husbands' time and energies to minimize loss of earnings. In other families, where there was less financial pressure, the response was different. Men abandoned their commitment to promotion, and the increased money and status it brings, and assumed a much greater involvement in family life than might otherwise have been the case.

It is interesting, in view of their reduced incomes and extra commitments, that so many families in the study managed to cope without running into serious financial trouble more often. A number of explanations can be offered, some more speculative than others.

The first, and perhaps most speculative, is that severe disablement in a child altered the financial relations of husbands and wives so that they co-operated in planning and decision-making more than they would otherwise have done, and more of the men's earnings were available for general family expenses than would normally have been the case. The distribution of money within the family in Britain is a relatively uncharted area and it is not possible to test these ideas using comparative data.[1] However the depth interviews produced a strong impression that the majority of these couples were very open and cohesive in their dealings about money. Men also frequently mentioned being less willing or able to keep back as much money for themselves as they would normally have done. The mother of a very hyperactive four-year-old boy gave this as their reason for being able to manage so well:

'We work together with money. We don't smoke, we don't drink. My husband hardly ever goes out – once a week for a drink. And if the bills come in we've got the money. We might not have much left over, but it's there. We ask each other about what we've paid, and we check up. . . . And we plan. He tells me his wage.'

There was also evidence of a level of support from relatives, particularly grandparents, which was possibly greater than if the child had not been disabled. Again, not enough is known of the general pattern and level of support from relatives at different stages of the family life-cycle to test whether these families had an unusual amount of help. In the present study financial support from relatives was greatest when children were young, and was often considerable. Going beyond the family itself, cash benefits were an important source of help, especially for families receiving the maximum amount available. Services in kind, such as incontinence equipment, free transport to school and assistance with housing adaptations again were an important buffer for the families who succeeded in obtaining them. Conversely, however, when such services were unreliable, discontinuity in the provision of help could lead to considerable extra expense. When school buses failed to arrive, for example, taxis had to be paid for.

Another, less speculative, reason for families managing without breakdown was that they became extremely skilled in their handling of money. There was overwhelming evidence from the survey and from the depth interviews of the care and precision with which finances were managed. Women mentioned knitting, sewing and mending much more than they would normally have done. Shopping patterns changed, with families more frequently buying in bulk whenever possible – especially items which the disabled child used heavily. It seemed that having a disabled child caused poorer families to assume budgeting patterns usually associated with more affluent, middle-class life-styles – buying in bulk from warehouses, shopping in bulk and freezing food and so on. Women whose child was incontinent mentioned constantly, and almost automatically, looking for cheap plastic pants, toiletries and trousers and stock-piling them. On the other hand, not all families were free to adjust their shopping patterns so as to minimize extra expense. Families with hyperactive, very dependent or immobile children often remarked that their normal shopping was dearer because they had to use local shops and were unable to shop around for bargains.

The depth interviewers were specifically asked to form their own judgments about families' budgeting skills.[2] For forty of the forty-eight families interviewed money management was judged to be very good. For sixteen of these the assessment was that it was exceptionally good. Two of the remaining families were under extreme stress because of the child's condition and their handling of money was haphazard and disorganized at the time. These budgeting skills had not always been there. Several families had found themselves in severe financial trouble at different times and had had to make conscious and painful efforts to learn how to manage their money. Particularly when parents were very young and the disabled child their first they found it difficult to learn to budget, especially when the child's condition was unstable or involved hospital admissions.

All the families in the study were asked whether the child's disablement had altered the way they managed their money or their financial priorities. Thirty-eight per cent of them said it had done so, in the ways shown in Table 7.1

*Table 7.1 Changes in the ways in which money is handled**

	No. of families	%
More saved – for the future, for major items or for emergencies	81	17
Disabled child's needs given priority	33	7
Have to be more careful with money because income lower or disabled child's costs high	43	9
Live from day to day now/don't plan	26	5
Unable to take on HP or other forms of credit	15	3
Other answers	11	2
Total no. mentioning any change = 185		
No. of families in the sample = 480		

*Families could cite more than one change.

It is interesting that so many families mentioned a need to save. It might have been expected that they would be less able to save than other families. It was not possible to compare families' savings with those of the control families. However, families in the depth interviews frequently mentioned both taking out extra life assurance so that a surviving partner could afford to stay at home to look after the child, and saving to have a reserve for emergencies. Clearly, the ability to do this depends on income: several families had nothing whatever to fall back on and no insurance. Table 7.1 also shows that, for some families, the child's condition had had the effect of making them *less* careful with money. This was particularly so when the child's prognosis was poor – as with this multiply disabled sixteen-year-old:

> 'We save less because we think for Michael's sake we have to do things *today*, as soon as we can. We've changed our life-style completely. Normally we would have had savings – have a little bit behind us. And I would never have anything unless I could afford it. But we couldn't afford this bungalow and we took the risk and had it. We plan less carefully with money and we talk together about it more.'

A third reason for families managing to cope with reduced

incomes and extra costs was that the presence of the disabled child created involuntary savings. Parents frequently mentioned restrictions on their social lives, which inevitably meant lower expenditure – on alcohol, meals out, entertainment and adults' clothing. The comparative data confirms that spending on alcohol and adults' clothing was lower among the families with disabled children. It is important to remember, however, that parents generally minded these restrictions on their social lives and felt that they increased the stress of caring for the child.

For many families economies were enforced, rather than involuntary. Social life, with its attendant expenses, was the most frequently mentioned item when families were asked whether the costs associated with the child's condition had forced them to economize on anything. Almost half of the sample said there were things they had been forced to cut down on or give up. The economies most frequently mentioned were on parents' social lives and clothes and family holidays.

Parents were very aware of differences between their own lifestyles and those of other families they knew – particularly as children grew up and those families began to buy new furniture for their homes, go out more and take holidays abroad or in hotels. This woman with a thirteen-year-old cerebral palsied daughter, whose husband's earnings were very low and who was unable to go out to work herself, reflect on how their lives were different from other people's:

'Yes, we are hard up because of Tracy. Because, if you are parents with two children, at our age you should be enjoying yourself a bit after struggling for sixteen years. You should be reaping the benefits a bit now, but we don't seem to be getting any further advanced than when we started. To go out, it's an effort. Not because we can't be bothered to go out, but financially. We haven't got the money to go out. Plus the only person we have to look after Tracy is my mum. And my mum is seventy now and Tracy is just too heavy for her. No one else seems to realize the tension you have. So we seem to row and bicker more. Clothes we can't have, or a couple of pints up the road. And we've had to pack up smoking. And make-up, hairdo's, that sort of thing. I have everything when it's *really* necessary for going out. I hear people say – my friend, for instance, "Oh, I couldn't *bear* to go into a chemist without coming out with some make-up or nail varnish." And I wonder how they do it. I think if I hadn't had to buy these things for Tracy I could buy odd things for myself. . . . And it's the whole family goes without. And holidays. We've never ever had a proper holiday. We go off for a day or two sometimes to a chalet his sister owns, at the end of the season, but even then we take our bare housekeeping money – no more. A box of groceries we take.'

For professional people the discrepancies could be just as great. The father of a severely disturbed seven-year-old deaf-blind child who caused a lot of extra expense said he often compared his standard of living to that of his colleagues at work (he was a graphic artist and part-owner of his firm):

'In the long run it's held us back by several years compared to them. They have things like colour TV, stereo units, second cars for their wives, foreign holidays, new kitchen units and fridge-freezers. We always seem to be last in getting things. Even with second children we're last! They've all had their second children four or five years ago. And I've got a lower mortgage than all of them. You see, they've all had wives who've been able to go out to work.'

For most families everyday living was less of a problem than accumulating money to replace large items like cars or furniture or for holidays, as with the parents of this thirteen-year-old boy with Down's syndrome:

'We never get holidays now. Seeing the seaside is just a day trip and that's it. We never go away to stay. And even in earlier years when we went away it was a caravan, not a hotel. But that's not really a holiday. It's six years since we went away at all. . . . And there would have been more money to spend around the house, outside and in, without a doubt. I would have had heating. Perhaps little conservatories built outside to stop the draughts and the wind and the rain battling in at the door. Money that I would have spent in general on the upkeep of the property outside and in, and to make it more comfortable. Perhaps the odd bit of furniture – like I could do with a small settee. Just little things I can't afford now.'

These alterations in life-styles and living standards encompass both day-to-day economies designed to keep families solvent and the longer-term effects of living on tight budgets with little margin for treats or saving for larger purchases. They helped to prevent families from running into major financial troubles. There were indications, however, that a number of families in this sample frequently did not manage to make income and expenditure balance, in spite of their budgeting skills and economies. Housing costs and fuel bills were frequently mentioned as causing problems and families described budgeting strategies which basically consisted of juggling with commitments so that one was met by defaulting on others:

> 'We always, all the time, rob Peter to pay Paul. . . . We manage with our food and that, but it's always a struggle finding money for our bills. When they come in something else has to be left to pay them.'
> (Mother of an eight-year-old severely mentally handicapped boy)

This type of budgeting strategy is well documented in the literature on family finances and budgeting patterns,[3] and is normally associated with low income. Among these families with disabled children money problems and the need for constant juggling with finances were not confined to the poorer families. There were indications that many families were stretched financially and that this was caused by the child's condition.

Seventy per cent of the parents in the sample said they worried about money and about not being able to cope financially. Eighteen per cent said that they were 'quite often' worried, 26 per cent that they were worried 'most of the time'. Thirty per cent of parents thought they were 'more' or 'a lot more' hard up than most people. Two-thirds of these families attributed their financial stress to the child's condition, though some were reluctant to identify the disabled child as the cause of their difficulties. One mother who consistently played down any effect her severely disabled spina bifida child had had on the family's life, said:

> 'Well, over the years I suppose we've had some expense, but I don't like talking about it. I don't like to *say* that she's cost me any more, because I wouldn't be without her. I feel guilty saying that she's cost me more money.'

Other parents, however, found it much less difficult to analyse the disabled child's effect on their finances and were able to be fairly dispassionate about the importance of money in creating or alleviating stress. The mother of a very disturbed, hyperactive and destructive fourteen-year-old, for example, said:

> 'It does cost more money. In damage alone over the years it must have cost us hundreds of pounds. She'd sit and systematically tear the pages out of her books, for example. And money *is* important, it eases the strain. We feel less financial strain now than we did a few years back. When Ann causes some damage *now* we don't think "Flipping heck, how are we going to afford to replace that." We just get on and forget about it. We were tight with money at one time and if that had gone on the whole family would have fallen through. With that added worry it must be terrible. . . . I really feel for someone who's the caring mum of a handicapped child in adverse conditions. I don't know what keeps them sane.'

It has been suggested, both here and in the previous chapter, that families with a disabled child are more likely to experience chronic financial stress or financial crises than other families with children. To explore whether these families had experienced such stress they were asked about the disabled child's effect on their finances in the previous year, using a number of indicators of financial stress. Table 7.2 shows the number of families reporting that their finances had been disrupted in various ways. Forty-one per cent had been affected in at least one of these ways.

Table 7.2 Signs of financial stress in the preceding year*

As a direct result of child's needs families have had to:	No. of families	%
Borrow money	105	22
Buy more on credit than they would otherwise	80	17
Delay paying bills	69	14
Spend money from long-term savings	67	14
Stop regular saving	56	12
Cash in or give up insurance policies	40	8
Total no. responding = 197		
Total no. of families in the sample = 480		

**Parents could give more than one answer.*

The commonest reason for financial stress was finding money to buy, repair or run cars, though general shortage of money was mentioned almost as frequently. The commonest ways of finding extra money were borrowing and buying things on credit that would normally have been bought for cash. Relatives and friends were the commonest source of loans, though almost half of the families in the sample had borrowed money from banks or finance companies and 14 per cent had borrowed money from several sources.

These or similar money problems will be experienced by many families with children. We cannot say whether they were more prevalent among these families. Even if they were not, severe disablement in a child must add an extra dimension to the stresses of living on an insufficient income. Paying fuel and other large bills late had become almost a regular way of managing money for some families in the sample. It remained a source of stress, however, particularly when mortgage or rent arrears built up to a worrying level or when the disabled child was very ill or stressful to care for. A women with a very frail cystic fibrosis child was extremely anxious and stressed because during a spell when her husband was on short time she had allowed mortgage arrears to build up. She was under pressure to clear them by the end of the local authority financial year, had been unwilling to worry her husband about money and could see no way of paying off the arrears. The very hard-pressed parents of a totally dependent quadriplegic spastic boy who was unable to go to school said that they were physically and financially exhausted, needing but unable to afford a holiday:

> Just at the moment I think we're getting to the end of our tether. . . . We both desperately need a holiday. We need something *doing*. You do really get desperate. And he can't concentrate on his work. . . . But you'd be amazed, on the other hand, how much happiness Stephen has brought us. He's a smashing lad.'

Three weeks after the interview the father had a major heart attack.

Sometimes, when families were very poor, the disabled child's needs could not be met, and this caused great distress to parents. Those who had been advised to keep a child warm or on a high-protein diet would agonize because they could not afford to do this when, for example, men were unemployed or on short time. Now and again the disabled child's health could appear to be directly threatened by a simple lack of money. These parents, for example, were unable to afford a taxi to get their spina bifida child to hospital quickly when it seemed that her valve had blocked:

'Last year when Kate was ill, it was a cold. But we thought it was her valve playing up. They said if she was drowsy and listless for two days we should bring her in. And that night she started to cry, and I'd never heard her cry like that. And we rushed out and couldn't get a taxi because we had no money and we had to get a bus. It was so frustrating. The bus went so slow. And we were thinking, "Look, she could be dying and we can't get her there." And that happened five or six times that year. It was terrible.'

It is almost certain that an ambulance would have been provided had these parents requested one. However both were under twenty at the time, were not sure whether this was enough of an emergency to justify using the ambulance service and did not, in any case, have easy access to a telephone.

Parents' views of the child's effect on their living standards

Parents were asked in some detail in the depth interviews how they felt about the disabled child's effect on their standards of living – what they minded most, how they coped with doing without things other people had, and how they made sense of having less money. Clearly, parents' responses to these questions will be bound up with their general philosophy of life and their expectations both of parenthood and of material progress. These and other factors will influence the meaning parents with a disabled child give to the child's disablement and to its effect on their own lives. Voysey and others have explored how parents with a disabled child interpret their situation and the complexities involved in reconciling ideas of normal parenthood with their own atypical experience.[4] In the light of such complexities the questions asked in these interviews may appear somewhat naïve. They did, however, elicit responses which pointed to ways of adapting and coping which were rational and coherent.

Many parents were unable to point to things they minded very much doing without. This was not because they were perfectly content with their lives but because, especially when the disabled child was older, they had become used to their way of life. They were unable to remember very clearly what life had been like before the disabled child was born; if they had no other children they had no strong idea of what life with a non-disabled child would have been like. The child's disablement was felt simply to have altered their lives so completely that it was difficult to think how it had been before:

> 'It's a different life and we've got used to it. . . . I think there was a time when we hadn't had Peter very long when we used to say, "I wish we had this, and I wish we had that", but I think you get to the stage where you don't think about it.'
> (Mother of a nine-year-old boy with spina bifida)

When asked directly what they minded sacrificing, then, the majority of parents said they had got used to and accepted the disabled child's effect on their standard of living. 'Accepting' in this way was, however, a deliberate strategy for survival rather than not noticing that there had been an effect. Parents frequently said that they refused to dwell on financial and other aspects of the child's condition because this was too depressing. They also liked to be able to present themselves to the outside world as coping, as these fairly typical responses indicate:

> 'You don't go sitting round thinking what you're going without. . . . You'd go mad. It's a question of facing up to facts and trying to live on a tight budget without having to go round crying on people's shoulders, saying you can't do this or can't do that – and at the same time put a face on it that gives the impression you're doing all right.'
> (Mother of a thirteen-year-old spastic boy)

> 'I think you like to make things look as normal as possible. I think you don't want to make things sound *too* bad. You like to feel you can cope. But it comes sometimes when you begin to wonder whether you *can* cope. Like last time he was in hospital.'
> (Mother of a four-year-old boy with a congenital heart defect)

Accepting also meant coming to terms with the probability that some things – like owning a house – might never be possible, and adjusting previous expectations:

'You do get used to things. I know the kind of life I'd like, the kind of house I'd like. But I can't see me buying a house. I accept the fact that we're not going to have what we thought we'd have – a reasonably furnished house. A more comfortable house. Possibly a car, that sort of thing. No way can we afford it.'
>(Father of a thirteen-year-old girl with a rare skin complaint, ichthyosis histerix)

This tough-minded willingness to accept and to get on and cope with the lot that had fallen to them was related, by some parents, to their general attitude to the risks of having children:

'We'd positively planned to have children, and accepted the consequences and the responsibilities of that. And if they happen to come out with funny-shaped feet and it costs you more then that's tough but you get on with it.'
>(Father of a profoundly deaf, hyperactive five-year-old)

Others were helped by the realization that there were other people in worse situations.

None of these strategies, however, precluded occasional wistful feelings or pangs of misery, when from time to time parents compared their own life-styles with those of other people they knew:

'You do think how things might have been. And the older you get the worse it becomes. People say you get used to it. You accept it, because what else can you do. But you don't really get used to it.'
>(Mother of a fifteen-year-old mentally handicapped girl)

Perhaps the kind of thing parents missed most was money for occasional treats – like being able to buy presents for each other from their own money. It was more usual, too, for husbands to point out what their wives had missed out on, and wives their husbands, than for either to dwell on their own deprivations. The mother of a cystic fibrosis child mentioned how much her husband minded the fact that since his whole wage went into ordinary living expenses his birthday present to her simply meant that the housekeeping was that much shorter that week. The wife of an accountant minded the fact that her husband had to have cheap shoes and chain-store suits when his professional colleagues wore leather shoes and hand-stitched suits.

An important way of making light of any financial deprivation of their own, or of the rest of the family, was to stress that the child's disablement had completely altered their priorities. His or her needs and quality of life took precedence over their pleasures – or, more accurately, meeting these needs had become a source of pleasure in itself. Unselfishness is one of the qualities expected of 'good' parents in our society; many of these families had cultivated it to an extent which must have left little room for even the smallest self-indulgence. If the disabled child was well and happy most other things could be coped with, as these parents of a four-year-old spina bifida child said:

> 'With us now Anna comes first before everything. She'd always come first. As long as we've got food to eat and Anna doesn't have to go into hospital for operations it's all right.'

Such views were frequently associated with a reluctance to acknowledge that the child's disablement had had *any* effect in case it appeared that the child was being blamed for this – either to the interviewer or within the family generally:

> 'I feel as though we're blaming this kid. . . . I don't want to attribute anything to David. I don't want anyone to feel that we've had to struggle through life because of David. He *has* been an extra cost factor, but he's well worth it.'
> (Father of an eight-year-old boy with Down's syndrome)

When there was any possibility that children might not live very long such feelings were, understandably, stronger and parents were conscious of trying to cram as much as possible into a short space of time. On the other hand, parents of hyperactive, destructive, non-communicating children had a much more difficult task in making sense of the child's effect on their money and general life-style. Constantly replacing damaged possessions could be very demoralizing and parents would sometimes opt for living with extremely old, shabby furniture in houses where everything breakable was removed or placed at a height, rather than watch things being destroyed. These parents' attitude seemed, on the whole, bleakly stoic, whereas parents whose children were able to communicate and were not destructive could derive pleasure from sacrificing to give the disabled child a better life:

> 'We think "Oh God, we've got to pay for that" when there's damage. But we don't dwell on it. We pay for it and we go on. . . . We've evolved a system, because money is not *that* tight, of paying for it and forgetting it. Otherwise we'd go crazy. . . . The only things we don't have, that a normal family would have, are nicer, more fashionable things for the house. A normal family would have replaced this suite ages ago. But we know that whatever we'd bought would have been ruined. And we feel that we'd be far more frustrated at a £400 three-piece suite being drawn on with biro than living with this one and hoping that people don't too much mind sitting on it.
>
> (Mother of a fifteen-year-old hyperactive girl)

The help that should be given to families with disabled children

Clearly, parents' views of the help that should be provided for disabled children and their families will be influenced by their own financial circumstances, by the financial impact and general nature of the condition, and by their previous experiences of seeking and obtaining help. Their views on the nature of individual and community responsibility for the care of dependent people will also be influential. It is not possible here to do full justice to the views parents expressed on these complex topics. We can only look briefly at whether parents thought they should have more help, why they felt they ought to have such help and what they saw as the most useful form it could take.

Cash benefits

All the parents with disabled children were asked whether they thought the government should give more help in cash benefits to families with disabled children. Fifty-eight per cent replied that more cash help was needed; 42 per cent that the amount currently given was adequate. These answers were not influenced by the amount already received in benefits, the exception being families receiving only higher-rate attendance allowances, significantly more of whom thought that more cash help was needed. It was suggested earlier (p. 97) that these families were inequitably treated, vis-à-vis families who received both higher-rate attendance allowances and mobility allowances. It is interesting that they should articulate, more than other groups, a view that cash help should be increased.

In the depth interviews parents who had given either answer were questioned more closely about what they had meant. Parents who had said existing cash help was adequate fell into four groups: those who were receiving the maximum possible amount in benefits; those where the financial impact of the condition was slight and covered by the benefits received; those who were in neither of these situations but who did not want to appear greedy; those who preferred any increase in government expenditure to be channelled into services rather than benefits.

The families who had said that more cash help was needed were more likely to be hard-pressed financially – because their incomes were low or the child's expenses heavy, or a combination of the two. They stressed that present benefits did not approach the amount lost in earnings. Where families were poor existing benefits, though helping them to cope, did not enable them to meet the disabled child's needs properly or improve the quality of his or her life. They also emphasized that the stressfulness of their lives meant that they needed money for holidays or regular outings. A small number of parents said that it was important that cash allowances from central government be increased to allow families to meet the disabled child's needs themselves with privacy and dignity. These parents resented constantly having to give information about what they saw as essentially private matters (their incomes and savings) in order to get help from local authorities.

Parents in both groups expressed ambivalence about the appropriate amount of cash help to expect. Even where they were firm that they needed more help parents would acknowledge that some of the responsibility was their own, that they were very grateful for the help they got and did not like to be seen as receiving money for having a disabled child.

'I don't like to ask for money. I don't see why I should. She's mine. I have to keep her. She doesn't belong to the government.'
        (Mother of a fourteen-year-old girl with spina bifida)

The rationale for government help

In Chapter 2, the case for providing financial help or compensation to disabled children and their families from public funds was argued from the perspective of the disinterested observer. We were interested to explore how this compared with what parents themselves saw as the rationale for government help. All the parents in the sample were asked whether they thought it right that families with disabled children should be given cash benefits and other forms of help and, if so, why. All but eleven families thought it right that they should receive financial help. As Table 7.3 shows, a wide range of reasons was given in support of this view. The largest group of parents identified the disabled child's special needs and extra costs as the reason, though these answers may have been influenced by the purpose of the study. The second

Table 7.3 *Parents' views of why the government should give financial help to families with disabled children**

	No. of families	%
A disabled child costs more to bring up than other children	157	32
It would cost the state more to keep the disabled child in care/hospital	113	23
Families need money to relieve stress	102	21
Because families cannot manage without help	98	20
Because parents' earnings are affected	66	14
To give the disabled child a better life	45	9
It is nobody's fault so families should not have to cope alone	36	8
We pay taxes and National Insurance to cover such contingencies	30	6
The child's handicap may be the result of vaccine damage or other failure of care by doctors	11	2
Other answers	61	13
Total no. responding = 469		
Total no. of families in the sample = 480		

*Parents could give more than one answer.

commonest reason given was the savings families with disabled children make for the government by caring for their children at home; the need for money to relieve family stress was the third. Only 4 per cent of parents saw their payment of National Insurance contributions and taxes in the past as the reason why they should be helped. These parents saw themselves, that is, as members of a welfare state, one of whose functions was providing for contingencies such as disablement in a child. A further 5 per cent gave the related reason that, because the child's disablement was no one's fault and could not be anticipated, his or her care should be a communal, rather than a private family responsibility.

It might be expected that views such as these would be associated with feelings of entitlement to help, rather than with feelings of guilt or shame. However the depth interviews indicated that only a tiny minority of parents had strong feelings of entitlement to help. The majority were defensive or deeply ambivalent about their dependence on the state or the community at large:

'No, I don't feel I have a right to it. But I don't see any reason why the government *can't* give us an allowance. After all, it's nobody's fault he was born handicapped.'
    (Mother of a nine-year-old boy with spina bifida)

'We believe people are responsible for each other. We're Christians, so that's what we believe. But it's a bit different, somehow, when it comes to taking money yourself from other people. Like when the attendance allowance came out at first, for example, we thought – why should they give us money? Lee's our responsibility.'
    (Father of an eleven-year-old mentally handicapped boy)

It was not uncommon for mothers, who usually cashed the child's benefits, to try and make sure that local people were not in the Post Office when they were cashed, or to feel that counter clerks disapproved of them for getting money for the child:

'Even now, I'll admit, when I go to the Post Office when I go in I get the feeling he's thinking "Hello, here's that scrounging bugger." When Marjorie [his wife] goes in for the attendance allowance she *crawls* in, because we have always to use one Post

Office. I'm not saying he does think that. He's charming. But I go in and because of my job I have to have reasonably smart clothes, and we've a biggish car. And I get the feeling he's looking. And I'd hate my colleagues to think I'm getting these. To them it's a state handout and you're a scrounger.'
(Father of an eight-year-old Down's syndrome boy)

Nor were these feelings entirely imaginary; several people said they had experienced hostile or envious remarks from neighbours about their being able to run a car or to have colour television because they had a disabled child.

Many parents found it difficult, then, to reconcile their guilt and embarrassment at getting money for something they would have preferred to be able to cope with alone, with a real need for help and a strong feeling that the job they were doing should be recognized by the community. They did not want to be seen as scroungers but could not do without help:

'Yes, with a handicapped child we feel we *should* get some help. But we just don't really like asking, or writing begging letters for charity. I would feel better if someone came and asked *us* is there any help we'd like, instead of us always having to chase somebody.'
(Father of a four-year-old brain-damaged girl)

A few families were more robust in their attitudes – a former shop steward, for example, now working on the management side of his firm, had a strong and coherent idea of the reciprocities involved in the fiscal and social security systems. In his capacity as a voluntary organizer of the local MENCAP society he spent a fair amount of time encouraging and helping other families to apply for benefits 'because it's their right'. Even he, however, felt uneasy about receiving cash help for himself:

'Do I feel as if I have a right to help? If I was talking about somebody else's child I would say yes. But for some reason you get some sort of inhibition because you're the person involved. God, I've been on soap boxes virtually, arguing socialist principles on things like this, and yet because it's my child I tend to be, to feel, embarrassed. And it's nonsense really. I'll fight and fight at city level for mentally handicapped children – or for someone else. I'll say, if I discuss it with another parent at the PTA, "You go and damn well get that, because you're entitled

to it." But when it comes to yourself, it's different. I feel the right exists, but I feel uncomfortable because I might be taking it from someone who needs it more than I do.'
(Father of a fourteen-year-old girl with Down's syndrome)

Time and again parents pointed to this paradox of being able to see other people as having rights to help which they did not themselves feel they had:

'I would tell anybody to ask for their rights. It's funny. And yet you won't do it for yourself. I mean, if I had a friend that had a child I would be only too willing now to say, "You get in for as much as you can." And yet I haven't done it myself. . . . I think myself, "Well, am I being greedy?" We don't practice what we preach.
(Mother of a nine-year-old boy with spina bifida)

The saving of institutional costs was frequently used as a way of resolving these internal tensions between need, entitlement and stigma – though feelings about the views of neighbours and friends were often unresolved:

'I think life is difficult enough *with* help, and I think we should have everything there is. It costs £60 a week to keep a child in a home, so if anyone will keep a child at home they should have all the help they can get. . . . And yet. Duncan used to go to a playgroup in the school holidays, in a minibus. They used to come for him, and I got to hear one of my neighbours had said – "She's getting paid for him and she doesn't have him." And that sort of thing affects you.'
(Mother of a nine-year-old Down's syndrome boy)

Parents were much more likely to talk of feeling that they were begging or scrounging by applying for disability benefits than of feeling they had a right to help. These feelings applied less often, on balance, to getting help through services, though they were still diffident about asking for help – particularly when a means test was involved.

It is not possible here to go beyond this sketchy account of what is a very complex subject. It is clear, however, that many of these families with disabled children, though completely convinced in principle of the appropriateness of help being given by the community, had not translated these general opinions into specific feelings of personal entitlement to help.

Cash or services?

When parents were asked what would be the most useful form of help for them at present more of them mentioned financial help than any particular service (see Table 7.4). However almost twice as many parents said that their most urgent need was for a service of some sort.

Table 7.4 The type of help that parents would find most useful at present

	No.	%
More financial help }	105	
Financial help with transport }	43	31
Someone to look after the child sometimes to give us a rest	90	19
Better education and training facilities	80	17
Better housing	54	11
Someone to give advice, information and encouragement	44	9
Better facilities for long-term care	30	6
Better aids and equipment	19	4
Better medical services	12	3
Cannot say	3	–
Total	480	100

In the depth interviews they were questioned in more detail about their preferences for different forms of help and whether, if they had to choose, they would prefer increased cash help or better services. Clearly both are needed. Our intention in posing the alternative was to find out more about parents' immediate priorities and about their views of different methods of assessment and service delivery.

In weighing up their preferences for cash allowances and services parents were influenced by the following factors:

Their incomes and the pressures the disabled child's special needs placed on their budgets. The poorest families and those where the child's everyday costs were high were more likely to say they preferred cash allowances.

Their own child's particular needs and their general concern for children with disabilities. This meant that even very poor families could conceive of foregoing increased financial help in return for improvements in specialist services for disabled children – or even, in the case of two families, for expenditure on programmes to prevent disablement.

The practical possibility of using a cash allowance to substitute for services. This depended, in turn, on the availability and cost of a market alternative and the extent to which this could be used without technical expertise. Special education, vocational training and relief care cannot easily be purchased; choosing aids is thought to need special knowledge. Hence, most families could not see cash benefits as an alternative way of obtaining these. The question was rather whether money should be devoted to these *or* to an expenses benefit. In the case of the services in kind provided by local authorities, such as incontinence aids, it was more possible to conceive of substituting cash.

Previous experiences of claiming. Families who had had bad experiences of claiming help from local authorities or from supplementary benefit offices were likely to stress the desirability of cash allowances as of right.

The depth interviews revealed that, where there was a possibility of substituting cash allowances for services in kind, the majority of parents preferred to be given an adequate amount of money to spend as they saw fit 'without red tape and interference'. They expressed a strong desire to minimize the frequency with which they had to be assessed for help, particularly by local agencies and particularly through assessments which involved means tests. They resented:

Having, time after time, to reveal details of their incomes and personal lives in order to get help which their child needed. (They were also unhappy that this information was on file and accessible and their confidentiality threatened thereby.)

Being assessed by people who often did not have a detailed knowledge of their child's condition and its effects – not least the effect of disablement on their finances.

Delays, poor communications and other occupational hazards of dealing with bureaucracies.

The overlap of the social work relationship with decisions about whether material help should be given.

These resentments were clearly articulated by the mother of a very dependent quadriplegic spastic boy who managed, with great difficulty, to keep up appearances and give the child a reasonable life, but whose social worker clearly thought the family in a much better position than his poorer clients and therefore not in need of help:

'When people come to the house. . . . How can you tell them that the things you have, and that you've struggled for and cut back on your own personal habits to provide, are to make a pleasant atmosphere and a pleasant appearance for Mark? And don't mean that you've plenty of money? But when they ask what you do for a living the axe seems to fall. You get a bit fed up. Do you know, it can tire you asking over and over again. . . . And everyone has a file. And you have to repeat your tale over and over again as you ask for everything. Every piece of equipment. And everybody seems to pry into what you might call your private business. And they *keep* so much private information about you. I mean, you want a little bit of private life, don't you. . . . We fought about these things once, but now we have less heart for doing it. I'm getting old and I'm getting tired and I'm getting to the point where I'd rather trail my feet and drag on alone rather than ask them.'

These views referred only to locally administered services in kind, such as help with housing adaptations or special equipment. Where the services in question were those for which there was no easy market alternative, or which could improve the quality of the disabled child's life even the poorest families said they preferred improved services to higher cash benefits. The parents of a fourteen-year-old Down's syndrome child, for example, said they would happily do without their attendance allowance if better long-term care could be developed.

Most people who expressed a willingness to forgo increased cash help for improved services tempered such sentiments with a degree of cynicism (or realism) about the extent to which such choices were really possible. In an ideal world, it was felt, it *would* be possible to sacrifice additional cash in return for an improvement in the quality of your disabled child's life. In the real world it was better to take what was going and do your best with it. And most people were living at income levels where extra money could make a real contribution to their lives, even though in some cases appropriate services might make a bigger contribution. It could free money currently spent on the child and generally increase the family's standard of living, or it could ease the difficulties of paying for larger items like cars and holidays, which many families could not easily afford at present. People who were better-off were aware, too, of how different their lives would be on lower incomes and hence aware of the importance of increased cash help for poorer families. The father of an extremely hyperactive child, whose wife was very stressed, described why he thought they should have more money and the contribution it could make to relieving family stress:

> 'I see now they're advertising in the paper for foster-parents for disturbed children, and they're paying them £36 a week. Now I think looking after Peter, who's our own, is a harder job. . . . I think *we* should get £36 a week. . . . Joan can drive, but in no way can I afford a car. Now if these grants were so good that they could enable her to buy a Mini, to be able to take Peter out, that would alter our attitude. The tensions would be a lot less. And that's the only way the government could help, apart from getting someone to come in two or three times a week to babysit for you. But if we had a higher allowance so that we could buy a car it would ease a lot of her tensions.'

Parents were also asked what, if all existing forms of help were scrapped and policy-makers were asked for guidance about what future help should be based on, they themselves would recommend. This question elicited a very strong response that family stress and strain was the factor that cash help should be built around. Parents, and especially mothers, should be compensated or paid for the stressful caring job they had assumed:

> 'In the case of a handicapped child the whole responsibility mustn't be laid with the parents. And if there's any hardship at all for any part of the family's work – earnings, spending or whatever – the government should help with it. And the

attendance allowance alone doesn't meet it. If we had more money – if I could earn more – perhaps my wife would find it less stressful. The attendance allowance doesn't nearly cover my earnings loss. If we had more money then we could have a decent holiday, save, have a *decent* car to take Joanna out. I think the government should consider the effect on *all* members of the family. Not just the husband. Probably he's in the best position of all because he can leave the four walls whereas the wife and other children can't. . . . There should be some money to compensate the other children, the other members of the family – compensation for stress or the environmental effect.'

(Father of a very hyperactive, deaf, blind and aphasic four-year-old girl)

Clearly, then, most families saw a role for increased cash help, though for some it took second place to improved services, while for others the idea of receiving large sums of government money for having a disabled child presented problems.

This chapter has been concerned with the overall impact of the child's disablement on families' living standards and with parents' expectations of help. Appendix II relates this discussion to the experience of one of the families in the study. In the following chapter the study's implications for the development of financial provision for disabled children and their families are discussed.

8 Conclusion

This book has been concerned with the financial costs of caring for severely disabled children at home and with the effect of these costs on families' living standards. Of the many ways in which severe disablement in a child affects their lives, its effect on the family's standard of living is unlikely to be the one which parents themselves identify as most important. Unless they are experiencing a financial crisis, the disabled child's health and well-being, physical burdens of care and worries about the future are all likely to take precedence. Nevertheless, as parents themselves recognized, money is an important factor in enabling them to cope more easily and to live well. When there are continual money worries the physical and emotional stresses of caring for a very disabled child become even more difficult to manage. When small pleasures that are routine for friends and acquaintances become unattainable luxuries the daily grind can at times seem overwhelmingly bleak.

And in very obvious ways money can ease burdens and relieve stress for a time: by making it possible to buy labour-saving equipment, take a holiday, replace a worn-out car or simply buy something new to wear. It is important, therefore, to establish the extent to which severe disablement in a child, in addition to the physical and emotional burdens it creates for families, penalizes them financially.

For the families in this study the financial impact of the child's condition was considerable and pervasive, affecting not only parents' earnings and expenditure on the disabled child but also expenditure on themselves and other children, the timing of financial decisions and the general management of money. Most of the time these constraints on incomes and on the way money had to be spent could be coped with, though living standards were lower than they would have been. Families coped better or worse according to their budgeting skills, the level and stability of their incomes, the disabled child's needs and the help available from relatives and statutory or voluntary agencies.

This stable coping pattern could be broken, however – by

urgent needs for things that could not be afforded, such as car repairs or house adaptations – or by hospital admissions. These were frequently associated with earnings loss, extra expenses and disruption of families' normal budgeting patterns.

The financial impact of disablement in a child probably increases with the severity of disablement. This could not be confirmed by the present study – largely because all the children in the study were severely disabled.[1] It *was* clear that the impact varied with families' incomes: as incomes rose both earnings loss and extra expenditure on the disabled child increased. This reflects the greater capacity of better-off families to divert money to the disabled child without greatly reducing the family's standard of living. The effect on poorer families' living standards is probably much greater, even though the absolute size of earnings loss or extra expense is smaller.

The financial effect also varied with the ages of the children in the family. Severe disablement in a child appears to hold families at a stage of the family life-cycle where they are poor. Severely disabled children typically remain very dependent for much longer than usual. Hence parents' earnings capacity is affected for longer and differences between the incomes of families with disabled children and other families increase as children grow up. Ironically, the child's condition also creates pressure for families to buy expensive items like cars and to move to larger houses sooner than they normally would. In a sense, then, severe disablement in a child holds families' incomes at the poorest stage of the family life-cycle while forcing them to assume expenditure patterns belonging to a later, and more prosperous, stage.

There are factors which mitigate these effects: adequate earnings, financial and practical support from extended families, and statutory support in cash and in kind. Parents also cope by becoming more efficient in their handling of money and by co-operating more in financial matters. Some families make involuntary savings because the child's disablement limits their ability to spend money – on family holidays or parents' social lives, for example. Even so, many families in this study lived in a state of chronic financial stress in which they were constantly worried about money and forced into a constant juggling of commitments and resources. When sudden demands for money arose, as when children were admitted to hospital, they had very little to fall back on. The psychological stresses of families who do not share in the prosperity of friends and relatives as children grow up should not be underestimated, particularly since the physical burdens of care may increase with time, rather than diminish. The majority of parents expressed the view that more cash help was needed by families with disabled children, though the more prosperous families indicated that their own needs could be met more satisfactorily through improved services. Comparatively few families, however, had strong feelings of entitlement to help.

It was argued in Chapter 2 that disabled children and their families *do* have rights to help. Parents are primarily responsible for their children but not completely so. A collective responsibility for the well-being of children also exists. The state intervenes in many ways to ensure that parents fulfil their responsibilities – if necessary removing children from their parents and assuming parental responsibilities and rights on behalf of society at large. In the case of children with disabilities this collective responsibility is even clearer – partly because disablement itself is often a by-product of technological developments which benefit the majority, and partly because society so strongly asserts its rights to uphold the disabled child's right to life – against the wishes of parents if necessary. Clearly, the burdens of care that subsequently arise do not belong only to parents. In discharging what are in part society's obligations they have a right to expect adequate support.

It is clear from this study that the financial costs of caring for severely disabled children at home are considerably greater than the existing level of support from cash benefits, services in kind and the Family Fund. The case for improving financial support is strong. However problems remain about the most appropriate way of providing the support parents themselves want – particularly when, as now, resources for new developments are extremely limited.

Particular difficulties arise in considering the relative priorities to be given to an improvement in cash help as against improvements in services. An increase in the amount of public money allocated to disabled children and their families is clearly justified. It is less clear that any extra cash should be devoted as a matter of priority to a cash benefit to compensate families for the costs of the child's disablement. Services might equally ease the burdens and costs of caring for a disabled child. Though most families in this study were financially affected by the child's condition, and some extremely hard-pressed, a desire for cash support did not take overwhelming precedence over a desire for improvements in support services for families and specialist services for the children themselves. A number of fairly poor families indicated a willingness to forego any increase in cash help for a guaranteed improvement in those services. The great majority of more prosperous families expressed a strong preference for improved services rather than an increase in the level of cash benefits – though there were occasional major items such as housing or housing adaptations for which financial help was needed. It should be stressed that in neither case were families referring to the help in kind currently provided by local authorities, usually on the basis of a means test. Any extension of help in kind dependent on financial assessment of this sort was universally rejected.

Ideally, improvements in cash benefits and in services provision should not be seen as alternatives. *Both* should be improved and the longer-term development of social security provision considered alongside the development of services for disabled children and the long-term future of the Family Fund. Bradshaw, for example, outlines how adequate support for disabled children and their families could be provided through a more generous and more coherent system of cash benefits; improved services provided through local agencies; and back-up discretionary help from the Family Fund.[2]

For the moment, such a package looks like wishful thinking. And even if resources were available, a pragmatic view of policy-making in Britain suggests that a rational approach to policies for disabled children, in which the merits of improved services are traded off against improvements in cash benefits, is unlikely to occur. Organizational factors within the DHSS and the separate responsibilities of ministers make it difficult to plan or to consider priorities between cash and services in this way. Morever current restraints on public expenditure, together with long-standing difficulties in improving services for particular client groups via independent local authorities, suggests that substantial improvements in services for disabled children are unlikely. Improving cash support seems both administratively and politically more feasible.

This study suggested a number of ways in which relatively small increases in government expenditure could greatly reduce the financial stress currently experienced by some families with disabled children and reduce inequities in current provision.

Conclusion 169

1 The qualifying age for mobility allowance could be reduced to two and its coverage extended to include children who, though technically able to walk, have severe problems in using public transport. (This would include, for example, mobile hyperactive mentally handicapped children, frail children and some children with sensory impairments.) Transport costs were a significant problem for parents in this study with children under five and older children not eligible for mobility allowance. Nine per cent of families in the sample said their greatest outstanding need was for help with transport; most of these families did not have mobility allowances. The Pearson Commission recommended in 1978 that mobility allowances should be extended in this way.[3] The detailed case for such an extension, together with an estimate of the cost, has been made elsewhere.[4]

2 The criteria for attendance allowance could be altered in three respects:

> By abolishing the six months' qualifying period before benefit becomes payable and adopting instead the principle used in mobility allowances where benefit is paid if the condition is likely to persist for a certain period. Families in this study frequently said that the greatest disruption of their finances occurred at the onset or diagnosis of disablement.
>
> By making attendance allowances payable from birth in the case of severe congenital impairments or illnesses. Costs and financial disruption in the first year of life can be very heavy – particularly hospital visiting costs and men's earnings losses. There is no statutory source of financial help before the age of two. Some of these conditions will have been corrected by the time the child is eligible for an attendance allowance.
>
> By abolishing the regulation that attendance allowances are not paid when a child has been in hospital for more than four weeks. Parents are encouraged by medical staff to visit for long spells daily and very often do. In the absence of help with travel costs and child-minding costs for other children the attendance allowance should continue to be paid. This restriction in fact affects a very small number of children but causes both hardship and resentment among the families who are affected.

The cost of these amendments would be fairly small since the number of children affected is not large in any except the first category. Even there the number of new applicants in any year is not large.

3 To ease cash-flow problems arising from the need to purchase consumer durables or move house sooner than would otherwise have been the case a system of interest-free loans or periodic grants, perhaps administered by the Family Fund, could be introduced.

4 The acute financial stress arising from hospital admissions should be reduced by making statutory funds available to hospital social work departments, particularly regional specialist centres and specialist children's hospitals. Help is available at present from the Family Fund but neither social workers nor parents are very aware of this and both seem confused about the Fund's criteria for helping.

5 Some financial help should be made available to the very small group of severely disabled children unable to attend school, either because they are too ill or because appropriate provision is not available.

Even with improvements such as these, a strong case remains for improving the general level of cash support to disabled children and their families through a new cash benefit. However the possibility of introducing a new benefit raises difficult questions about its objectives. Should the aim be to compensate for parental earnings loss or to help with the disabled child's extra costs? Should the focus of any new cash help be the disabled child or the family – a major gap in provision at present is in support or compensation for the stresses experienced by parents and other members of the family in caring for very disabled children? Should the priority be to prevent hardship in the poorest families, where the disabled child's effect on living standards is greatest, or to compensate families at all income levels for the difference the child's condition has actually made to their living standards? Questions like these inevitably draw attention to the lack of clarity about objectives that characterizes social security provision for disablement at present. They would be easier to resolve in the context of planning a coherent and comprehensive scheme of income maintenance for disablement in general, in which disablement in children was explicitly addressed.[5]

Ultimately such questions will be resolved, if at all, by political and other value judgments as much as by rational considerations. For the moment it is possible to consider the possibilities for a new cash benefit in a more immediately practical way – that is, by trying to decide what would meet the greatest need, is easiest to assess and administer and does not prejudice progress towards a more adequate and coherent system of cash support for people with disabilities.

This study suggested the following options for a new cash benefit for severely disabled children. (Only one of these options is assumed to be a possibility at present, though all three might ultimately be elements in a disability income.)

A benefit to help with extra expenses.
A benefit to compensate for parental earnings loss.
A benefit to compensate the disabled child and other family members for the restrictions and stresses of severe disablement.

An expenses benefit

The introduction of a general expenses benefit of £4 a week (at 1978 prices) was recommended by the Pearson Commission.[6] Such a benefit could easily be justified by this study's findings. However it would be difficult to design appropriate criteria for an expenses benefit. The findings of this study suggest that no single criterion would identify all the children whose disabilities warranted an expenses benefit. Nor would it be easy to identify children with higher and lower costs. A benefit set at one level would give some children too much and others not enough, but there seems no easy way of resolving this. We found no clear relationship, for example, between the severity of the condition and the level of extra expense – partly because what is spent depends, in the end, on the amount of money available.

This is not to say that it would be impossible to design workable criteria for an expenses benefit. The criteria for benefits are in general fairly crude tools for identifying a target population. Rather than looking for one precise criterion it might be preferable to base eligibility for an expenses benefit on a number of criteria. These could include receipt of attendance or mobility allowance, the presence of particular diseases or impairments, being at a special school, and so on. An expenses benefit, paid at one level, could be awarded if any of a number of conditions were met and could be paid as a supplement to child benefit.

An earnings-replacement benefit

Given the difficulties of designing simple criteria for an expenses benefit it might be preferable to opt, instead, for a benefit to replace earnings lost by the child's main carer – usually the mother. This type of benefit has the advantage of being easier to administer since employment status is relatively simple to assess. The greater earnings loss of women with older children might be recognized by tying the level of benefit to the age of the disabled child or the youngest child in the family.

There are three ways in which earnings lost by women caring for a disabled child could be compensated. First, the coverage of invalid care allowance could be extended to include married and cohabiting women. Second, a new benefit for carers could be introduced, set at a level closer to average earnings. Recent discussions arising from the Green Paper on the Taxation of Husband and Wife suggest a third possibility – that the married man's additional tax allowance be abolished and the revenue gained used to improve support for all families with young children. Home responsibility payments could be made to women who did not go out to work because they were caring for young children. These would clearly be a useful way of directing financial support to families with disabled children and could continue to be paid as long as the mother did not go out to work.[7]

A carer's benefit paid only to women who do not go out to work poses two main problems. First, it does nothing for women who do go out to work but who work fewer hours and earn much less than they would have done. Second, in terms both of relief from isolation and personal fulfilment, many women with disabled children would prefer to go out to work rather than receive a benefit for staying at home. The needs of these women would perhaps be better met by making it possible for them to go out to work – probably part-time. These problems are not insoluble. A taxable benefit for carers, set at a realistic level, would go some way towards compensating earnings reduced because of caring for a dependent. If combined with increased flexibility in men's working hours and the provision of relief care it could enable parents who wanted to do so to combine caring for a disabled child with work outside the home.

A compensatory benefit

There are strong arguments for such a benefit – not least the fact that so many families in this study identified compensation for family stress and the restrictions imposed on the child by disablement as an outstanding gap in provision at present, and one which should be filled as a matter of urgency. A compensatory benefit, based on the child's disablement, would avoid the problems involved in making additional cash assistance dependent on a woman's not going out to work. Designing criteria and assessment methods for such a benefit might be difficult, however. The criteria currently used in the industrial injuries scheme offer one possible model. They are already used in assessing eligibility for compensation for vaccine damage and will be used in assessing eligibility for the new severe disablement allowance.[8] It is likely, however, that these criteria would need to be modified if they were to be used to assess children suffering from a wide range of disabling conditions which impose very different stresses on family life.

On balance, the arguments in favour of a benefit to compensate for women's loss of earnings outweigh those in favour of the other options. The present study confirms that women's earnings make a significant contribution to their families' living standards. Among this sample of families with disabled children those where women were not in paid employment were worse off, at all income levels, than other families with disabled children as well as their FES counterparts. A benefit to compensate for loss of women's earnings would help to redress this inequality and would also help some of the poorest families with disabled children. Perhaps even more importantly, such a benefit would be an important step towards formal recognition of the value and importance of the care married women increasingly provide for dependents on behalf of the community and which is completely unrecognized at present. As this study has shown, the psychological and financial costs of caring are very high. Commitment to finding ways of sharing them is long overdue.

Conclusion

Improvements in financial support for disabled children and their families have been postponed in the past because of lack of evidence that disablement in a child penalizes families financially. That evidence is now available. It has been demonstrated clearly that severe disablement in a child has a substantial impact, both on families' incomes and on their expenditure patterns. There are a number of options for improving financial support for disablement in children, each with its own justification. The one option which has no justification at all is to do nothing.

Appendix 1
Research methodology

I Sample size

It had been anticipated that a comparative study of families' incomes and expenditure patterns, yielding statistically significant results, would involve large samples and be a costly exercise. A necessary first step was to calculate the sample sizes needed to produce results clear enough for policy purposes. This involved discussing with the DHSS the sizes of the differences in income or expenditure that would be useful in making decisions about future cash benefits. The sample sizes needed to be sure that differences of that order could not arise by chance were then calculated and various possible methods for the study costed. This was done in consultation both with the OPCS and with Professor Graham Kalton, then acting as a statistical consultant to Social and Community Planning Research Ltd (SCPR).

This showed that in order to obtain statistically significant differences in average expenditures on a wide range of commodities, of a size useful for policy purposes, very large samples would be needed. For example, to ensure at the 99 per cent level that a difference of £1 a week in the two samples' average total expenditures had not arisen by chance a sample of 9,577 families with a disabled child would be needed. For a difference of £2 a sample of 2,594 would be required. To ensure that a difference of £2 a week in the samples' average expenditures on, for example, durable household goods was significant at the 99 per cent level a sample of 1,177 families with a disabled child would be needed. For comparisons *within* the disabled sample (assuming a sample size of 1,177 and cell sizes that were equal and equal to 100) differences of £15.30 or £11.60 in average weekly expenditure on durable household goods would have to be observed for the difference to be statistically significant at the 99 and 95 per cent levels respectively.

These calculations suggested that for a comparative study, yielding statistically significant results across the full range of expenditures, a sample of around 7,000 families with disabled children would be required. To obtain a large enough control group would require between 18 months and 2 years of the FES. The geographical spread of the disabled children and the consequent impossibility of clustering interviews meant that fieldwork costs would be very high. The cost of a study based on these sample sizes was estimated, in 1976, at a minimum of £350,000. The cost of such a large-scale survey was judged by the DHSS to be disproportionately expensive, measured against the likely value of the results. It was decided to mount a much smaller study.

A sample size of around 500 families with a disabled child was decided on. This was the largest number compatible with managing the complex fieldwork operations of the FES. It was, at the same time, the smallest number that would allow us to meet DHSS preferences for the study to cover a wide range of disabling conditions and allow the effects both of the condition and of families' incomes on the costs of disablement to be investigated.

Clearly, a sample of this size would not yield the robust, statistically significant findings produced by a study of 5-7,000 families with a disabled child. However, as noted in the text, sampling errors could be reduced by limiting the coverage of the study and by matching the samples on important variables. For some variables this could be done at the sampling stage; further matching could be carried out at the analysis stage.

II Matching the samples

It was necessary, first, to decide whether the FES sample should be matched to the Family Fund sample or vice versa, and second, to decide which variables to match on.

It was decided to match the sample of families with disabled children to the FES sample. This decision was taken because the Family Fund population could not be assumed to be representative of the general population of families with disabled children. Since the FES is representative of the general population of families with children it made more sense to match the families with disabled children, in important respects, to the FES sample. In this way we would be able to test whether the incomes and expenditure patterns of our sample of families with disabled children differed from those of a representative sample of families without a disabled child. (We would not, however, be able to extrapolate from this to the general population of families with a disabled child.)

The choice of variables to match on was influenced by three factors.

1 The information available from the Family Fund.
2 Evidence that the variables on which matching was proposed influenced expenditure.
3 The need to match in such a way that the effect of disablement on expenditure would not systematically be removed.

The Family Fund had information which would, in principle, allow matching on seven variables: region; social class; family composition; tenure; mother's employment status; father's employment status.

FES produces tabulations on all of these and all can have an effect on families' incomes and expenditure patterns. Some, however, may also be affected by the presence of disablement in a child – whether a woman is in paid work, for example, or the kind of house a family occupies. To match the sample on such variables might remove an effect of disablement. It was decided, therefore, to match the samples only on variables which were unlikely to be affected by the child's condition. In practice this came down to region and class.

There was a strong case for matching the samples on family composition at the sampling stage – that is, for mirroring the FES distribution of families with different numbers and ages of children. In practice this was impossible. First, Family Fund information quickly goes out of date so that by the time our sample was drawn children would be older and families bigger. Second, our matching had to be based on the FES for 1975, the latest available FES data. While major differences were unlikely to arise between 1975 and 1978 there might well be differences in the number and ages of children. Differences in family composition would, therefore, have to be adjusted at the analysis stage.

The age-structure of the disabled children had to be adjusted in one respect at the sampling stage. This was to attempt to counter the under-representation of children under five in the Family Fund population – the result both of Family Fund policy and of the time taken for some disabling conditions to become apparent. The age-structure of children in the disabled sample was matched to that of the general population of children under sixteen in England. Even so no disabled children under two were included in the study.

One further way in which the samples had to be matched was in the timing of fieldwork. Incomes and expenditure patterns vary over the year, the variation depending on changes in earnings and benefit rates, seasonal and regional price variations and inflation. FES draws its sample to take care of this by ensuring an even flow of interviews over the year.

We aimed to match that flow as far as possible. Fieldwork was restricted to two quarters of the FES, partly to restrict the amount of seasonal variation in incomes and expenditure patterns. It had been calculated that using the first two quarters of the year would give us a control group of around 700 FES families. In the event, as noted in the text, the timing of interviews differed slightly from that of the FES but not enough to have a significant impact on differences in earnings or prices.

III The method of drawing the sample of disabled children

Sampling frame

Families for the study were selected from the 41,449 families who had applied to the Family Fund by the end of September 1977. These families' records were physically stored in the Fund's York headquarters. The Family Fund data bank, stored on the University of York computer, contained information on important characteristics of the child and the family.

Criteria for the study

It was important that the number of successfully completed interviews be as near 500 as possible. The study's geographical coverage was therefore restricted to England and the composition of participating familes to single tax units containing two parents and no more than three children under sixteen. The disabled child was to be under sixteen on 1 January 1978 and living permanently at home. There were 14,193 records meeting these criteria at the time the sample was drawn and where, in addition: (a) the family's social class was recorded; (b) the family had been helped by the Family Fund.

Stratification

The sample was to be stratified by region (9 groups), social class (2 groups – non-manual and manual) and age of the disabled child (3 groups). This stratification produced 54 sample cells. The proportions used for the stratification were based on special tabulations of the 1975 FES data.

Drawing the sample

The sampling frame was divided into the 54 cells required by the stratification. The required number of families was drawn from each cell using random numbers, the full records of each family drawn being scrutinized to check that all the study criteria were met.

Response

To achieve the target quota it was necessary to estimate the likely response rate at the outset to ensure that a sufficiently large number of families was asked to participate. A pilot carried out in Birmingham indicated that 684 families would have to be approached to yield 500 successful interviews. The number was high, partly because families were likely to have moved and partly because their circumstances might have changed since the time they applied to the Fund so that they no longer met the study criteria. (Family Fund records are not updated.) There was reason to think that response might be much lower in other parts of the country where families are more mobile. Response was therefore monitored throughout the study so that more families could be approached if necessary. Dividing the sampling frame into 54 cells and using random numbers to select families allowed families not interviewed to be replaced by others who met the criteria for the study. In fact considerably more families had to be contacted (841 in all) than the pilot figures had suggested – particularly in Greater London and the South-East where families move more frequently.

IV The social class distribution of the two samples

At the sampling stage matching could only be attempted on a broad non-manual/manual split. This was because the Family Fund data are coded using the Registrar-General's classification of occupations while the FES uses an eight-point classification based on, but not identical to, this classification. The apparent relationship between the two systems is shown in Table A.1.

Table A.1 Relationship of FES occupation groups to the Registrar-General's classes

Registrar-General's classification	FES classification
Social class	Occupation group
I	1 Professional and technical workers
II	2 Administrative and managerial workers
	3 Teachers
III Non-manual	4 Clerical workers
	5 Shop assistants
III Manual	6 Skilled manual workers
IV	7 Semi-skilled manual workers
V	8 Unskilled manual workers

It was ascertained from the 1975 FES that for households in England with children the ratio of non-manual to manual workers was 35:65 per cent. This ratio was matched for the sample drawn from Family Fund records.

This matching process was successful according to the Family Fund coding of class. However in the course of the survey the occupation group of the head of household in families with a disabled child was coded according to the FES occupation group classification. Subsequently the proportions of men in the two samples in non-manual and manual occupations was found, surprisingly, to be significantly different (see Table A.2).

Table A.2 Social class distribution – based on head of household's occupation as recorded in the survey

Social class	Families with a disabled child		FES control	
	No.	%	No.	%
Non-manual	117	25	256	38
Manual	352	75	426	62
All households	469*	100	682	100
$X^2 = 19.5$	df = 1		$P < 0.001$	

*This total excludes unoccupied heads of households.

More precisely, 64 families coded as non-manual by the Family Fund were coded as manual on the FES classification; 18 families coded as manual by the Family Fund were coded as non-manual on the FES classification.

Some of these differences may reflect changes in occupation between application to the Family Fund and this study. There were two other reasons for the disparity. First, differences were found in the way the two classifications coded certain occupations as non-manual or manual. Police constables, for example, are coded as skilled manual workers by the FES but as skilled non-manual workers in the Registrar-General's classification. Second, detailed investigation of a sample of cases showed that the Family Fund coding of social class was inaccurate in some cases. Because sufficiently detailed information was unavailable to the coder, foremen and supervisors were in some cases wrongly classified as non-manual workers.

This difference in the samples' occupational structures had significance for the comparison of men's earnings. Since non-manual workers' earnings are higher, in general, than those of manual workers any difference observed in the samples' average earnings might simply reflect the different proportions of men in non-manual and manual occupations. For this reason comparisons were restricted to men in the same occupation groups and to men in non-manual and manual occupations rather than comparing men's earnings for the samples as a whole. A reweighting exercise was also carried out to ascertain how far differences in men's average earnings reflected the samples' different occupation structures.

Table A.3 shows the proportions of men in the two samples in each of the eight FES occupation groups. Weights were calculated by dividing the proportions in the FES control, for each occupation group, by the proportion of men in that occupation group with a disabled child. The resulting weights showed that there were substantially fewer men with a disabled child in the professional, administrative and managerial, and teaching groups. To obtain a reweighted average earnings figure for the families with a disabled child each man's normal weekly earnings were reweighted to the occupational structure of the FES control.

Had the distribution of earnings been very similar in each of the eight occupation groups reweighting would have resulted in a very similar average earnings figure for the two samples. However

Table A.3 Weights and weighted normal weekly earnings of men with a disabled child

Occupation group	Families with a disabled child % of sample	FES control % of sample	Weights
Professional and technical	5.9	14.2	2.4
Administrative and managerial	7.6	14.2	1.9
Teachers	2.0	4.3	2.2
Clerical	8.1	5.1	0.6
Shop workers	0.7	0.6	0.9
Skilled manual	46.4	39.2	0.8
Semi-skilled manual	24.8	19.3	0.8
Unskilled manual	4.4	3.1	0.7
Total number	407	607	
Original mean weekly earnings of the men with a disabled child	- £83		
- Weighted mean weekly earnings	- £84		
Mean weekly earnings of men in the FES control	- £92		

these distributions were obviously different. As Table A.3 shows, even when their occupation structure was reweighted to that of the FES the average earnings of the men with disabled children were still £8 a week less than those of the control. Hence the difference observed in the two samples' average earnings was not primarily due to their different occupation structures but to real differences in earnings between men in similar occupations.

V Diseases/disorders/injuries of the disabled children

The coding of the disorders affecting children who are severely disabled is complex as a child may suffer from several disorders. Table A.4 lists the principal disorders suffered by the children in the sample according to the disease classification developed by the Family Fund Research Team for coding applications to the Family Fund.

Table A.4 Diseases and disorders of the children in the study

	No.	%
Cerebral palsy	86	18
Mental subnormality	114	24
Down's syndrome	40	8
Spina bifida and hydrocephalus	30	6
Spina bifida	38	8
Deafness	17	4
Epilepsy/convulsions	15	3
Named syndromes	14	3
Muscular dystrophy	12	3
Microcephalus	15	3
Hydrocephalus	11	2
Suspected vaccine damage	4	1
Meningitis	5	1
Heart disease	8	2
Autism	5	1
Other central nervous system diseases	11	2
Maternal rubella	6	1
Werdnig Hoffman/muscular atrophy	5	1
Cystic fibrosis	4	1
Congenital defects of bladder, etc.	3	1
Other bone diseases	5	1
Tumours, Hodgkins disease, etc.	3	1
Brittle bones	3	1
Other physical malformations	4	1
Cretin/thyroid	1	0.2
Other blood diseases	2	0.4
Tuberose sclerosis	2	0.4
Renal disease/failure	2	0.4
Congenital defects of alimentary tract	2	0.4
Blind/vision defect	3	1
Skin complaint	2	0.4
Rheumatoid arthritis/Still's disease	2	0.4
Haemophilia	1	0.2
Head injury	2	0.4
Arthrogryphosis	2	0.4
Dwarfism (achondroplasia)	1	0.2
All disorders	480	100.0

Appendix 2
Case study: Andrew Cole

Andrew was fifteen at the time of the study and one of the most severely disabled children in the sample. He was quadriplegic, spastic, had no speech, was totally incontinent and was bronchitic. He also had an inoperable hiatus hernia which caused frequent vomiting. His hernia had led to a great deterioration in his health during the preceding twelve months and his parents had been told that he would probably not live beyond the next two years. He was not mentally handicapped, fully comprehending what was said but able to communicate his feelings or wishes only by grunts and whines. He could be extremely demanding, vocalizing continuously and loudly until his wants were met. Andrew was present throughout the interview, and both parents frequently, and apparently automatically, went to him to turn his head or move his limbs. At one point he vomited quite violently, although this was anticipated and bowl and handfuls of kitchen roll were at hand. He was clearly a considerable burden since he was totally dependent and unable to sit up unsupported. His family seemed, however, to have built their lives around him, without too much thought of the strain until the last few months and his deterioration.

The Coles lived in a pleasant private residential estate, of predominantly semi-detached bungalows. They had moved there five years before and chose both the bungalow itself and the district with Andrew in mind. They had converted the bungalow by extending the roof to the rear to add two extra bedrooms. The home was extremely comfortable and tastefully furnished within the family means.

Mr and Mrs Cole were in their late forties, and were responsible, sensible and extremely caring parents. They had been married for eleven years before adopting Andrew. His disability was not diagnosed until afterwards when there seemed to have been an attempt to take him from them – without success, as the adoption was then legal. Peter was conceived almost simultaneously and born within ten months. The couple then adopted

Anna as a baby. Both Peter and Anna were healthy, well adjusted and happy children who were very fond of Andrew.

Mr and Mrs Cole saw Andrew very much as their own responsibility, and were embarrassed by their inability to care for him without external help. To compensate their acknowledged guilt feelings about drawing mobility and attendance allowances, they both did voluntary work – Mr Cole on the committee for the Spastics' Society and his wife as helper at a playgroup for under-privileged and handicapped children. They were extremely concerned that colleagues and friends should not discover their receipt of allowances for fear of adverse reactions. Their financial circumstances appeared to be a very sensitive area. Consequently they had not received all the help they might have with the extra costs incurred by Andrew because of their unwillingness to disclose their circumstances.

The financial consequences of Andrew's disablement

1. Work and earnings

Andrew's mother was unable to work at all although she would normally have done so by now. The reasons for her being unable to work were: it took a very long time to get Andrew dressed and fed in the mornings; there had to be someone at home as soon as he returned from school, and when he was away from school ill or in the school holidays; her nights were so disturbed that she would be unable to cope with a job (she was regularly up four or five times in the night); she needed the day to organize things for the rest of her family. She had previously been a statistics clerk with the Electricity Board and would currently have been able to earn £3,000 a year in that job.

Mr Cole's work had also been affected. The main effect he saw was loss of promotion from being unable to move around the country to his firm's offices in other districts. He was unable to move because of the lack of specialized facilities for Andrew in many places. He thought he had also been held back by having to abandon his professional accountancy studies because he could not attend evening classes, nor could he go away on his firm's residential training courses. (Andrew was too heavy for his wife to handle alone for such a period.) He estimated that he would normally have been earning £1,500 a year more. At that time Mr

Cole saved a week of his annual holiday to take Andrew to hospitals, doctors, dentists, etc. Also since Andrew could no longer go away on holiday his father took one day a month off so that he and his wife could go out together. This was also time from his annual leave. Between both parents, then, there was an estimated earnings loss of £4,500 a year, assuming that Mrs Cole would have been working full-time.

II Day-to-day costs

Andrew's condition caused considerable extra expense which arose from:

Incontinence He was doubly incontinent and the Coles received no help from the Area Health Authority. They estimated that they spent £5.94 a week on items for incontinence and general medical purposes:

Large-size nappies	£12.15 per annum
Plastic pants	£ 2.00 a month
Creams, Calamine and Germolene	£ 4.00 a month
Disinfectant	£ 2.00 a month
Lavatory paper	£ 2.00 extra a month
Cotton wool	£ 1.00 a month
Kitchen roll	£ 4.20 a month
Aerosol sprays	£ 2.80 minimum a month
Laxatives and suppositories	£ 1.20 a month
Herbal remedies and cough medicines for bronchitis	£10.50 per annum

(The costs are given mainly in monthly terms because the shopping was done monthly.)

The Coles were very unclear about what help they could get with incontinence equipment and no one had offered help. Some of the items listed above are used not only for incontinence but also for Andrew's dribbling and vomiting.

Clothing and shoes Overall the Coles said they spent much more than they would expect to on Andrew's clothing. This was partly from his incontinence and dribbling. It was also because the rigidity of his body meant clothes tore easily when he was being dressed and undressed. He had to have special shoes made because his feet were long and narrow and he had to have shoes that opened all the way to the toe so that his parents could make sure his toes were not curled, which caused very painful cramp. They could not put a figure on the extra cost of Andrew's clothes and shoes but said they spent at least three times as much on them as they did on his brother's. Bedding was also worn out because his incontinence caused extra washing.

Fuel They used extra fuel for three reasons: extra washing and baths; Andrew felt the cold because of his immobility; they were up in the night a great deal and had to keep the house at a bearable temperature. (They also kept lights on in the hall all night.) They were aware of switching their central heating on earlier in the year than other people, keeping it on later in the year and keeping it on in the night when most people switch it off. Mrs Cole tried to economize by not using the central heating during the day.

Transport It was entirely impossible for Andrew to use public transport. Because his wheelchair was so big he needed a big car in which he sat in the front seat in a reclining position with the chair in the back. Two adults were needed to get him out and about. The Coles said such a large car used extra petrol and cost more in maintenance. They did not feel their actual mileage was much higher than it would have been. Though the mobility allowance was helpful with petrol, running costs and repairs, replacing their car was a major worry. (One *indirect* transport cost was the 20 miles a day Mr Cole travelled to work, having moved to the bungalow on Andrew's account.)

Recreation The Coles said they spent more than they would have done because there was so little Andrew could do himself. He was not mentally handicapped so they felt a responsibility to try and keep him stimulated. For example, they had bought an expensive music centre and bought lots of records and tapes for him. They had also bought a television set for his room, which was one way of giving *them* some relaxation. That expense, however, may have been balanced by their not spending on things like bikes and social life for him. They were asked whether they bought things to compensate Andrew and said not – that there was practically nothing you could compensate him *with*. However they were aware of a fair amount of compensatory spending on their other two children because of the restrictions on their lives – fewer outings and no spontaneity in them, no proper family holidays, less parental time and so on. So their parents tended to buy them the things they wanted: badminton rackets, bicycles, school holiday trips, etc.

Telephone calls   Their phone was originally installed on account of Andrew, because of having to ring school, hospitals, ambulances and so on. They still made use of it a lot for those reasons, and reckoned that about half their local calls were made on his account. They tried, in consequence, to economize on their own calls.

III. Capital costs

These again had been expensive – the biggest costs relating to housing and house adaptations.

House moves   Their house move was not because of Andrew but because of work reasons. However the house they moved to was chosen because it was a bungalow and therefore more suitable for him. It cost about £2,000 more than a semi-detached house would have done, and was ten miles further away from Mr Cole's work than the nearest house that was otherwise suitable.

Structural alterations   They had made the following adaptations:

   Additional bedrooms – to give Andrew a ground-floor bedroom of his own.
   A patio window – to give him easy access to the garden.
   Ramps – for easy access to the house and garden.
   Enlarged the kitchen – to make more room for manoeuvring his big wheelchair.
   Tarmac'd the driveway – because the wheelchair caught on the pebbles.

They approached their local Social Services Department for help with these adaptations but after being 'messed about something shocking' were told they had to be means-tested for anything that cost over £100. They refused to be means-tested and asked for £100-worth of help but were refused that. In the end only the ramps were fitted free. The remaining adaptations, which cost £2,100, were paid through a bank loan, so the true cost, after interest, would have been in excess of £2,500.

Equipment This was mainly supplied by the DHSS and the Social Services Department. Andrew had: 2 wheelchairs; a major buggy; calipers; a commode; a hoist to lift him on to the commode; bath aids. All were supplied free. The Coles had paid only for a lightweight buggy, which cost £25. (At the time the DHSS would not allow them to have three wheelchairs so they had to return their DHSS buggy.)

Special furniture They had bought:

	When	Cost
Special cushions for Andrew to support himself in bed	1978	£ 9
A special bed-side cabinet (made by his father)	1977	£10
A sun lounger, umbrella and parasol	1976	£20
Sheepskins to prevent pressure sores – they had bought several	1970 on	£10–£15 each

Other capital costs

A trailer for all his equipment	1976	£500 (paid for by the Family Fund)
Replacement of automatic washing machine through excessive wear	1974	£150
Frequent replacement of furniture damaged through incontinence	–	Could not estimate cost

Coping with the costs

The Coles received the maximum disability benefits – worth £21 a week at the time of the study. For large items they borrowed from the bank. They were very good managers of their money. Even so they had to cut down on things – principally the parents' clothes and social lives. Some of their economies had become involuntary, since Andrew's condition meant they were unable to go out much or go on holiday. They did not save at all but had a small amount saved for emergencies which they referred to as their 'sanity money'.

To summarize, Andrew's condition had created considerable extra costs. Because of Mr Cole's fairly high income they had usually had sufficient margin to absorb these without discomfort. Their problems arose with larger capital costs or when they had spells of expense, as when Andrew was in hospital for almost a year and visiting costs were high. (In that period they had exhausted their savings entirely on hospital visiting costs.) They dealt with large capital costs by borrowing from the bank and spreading the cost over several years, though this could create problems. Part of the reason for their bearing so much of the costs themselves was simply lack of information about what help was available. In addition their pride and independence meant they preferred to work like this rather than to submit to what they saw as an invasion of their privacy. The benefits they received certainly contributed to their ability to cope. The Coles had very interesting views on social security and the kind of help that would be most useful to them, as compared to poorer families. They thought that *they* could manage but that poorer people needed additional help. Even acknowledging those needs they wondered whether in the long run it would not be more helpful to invest any spare money in services – especially services to reduce the psychological strain on the whole family. They realized, however, that their views were very influenced by their own circumstances and that poorer people would probably prefer a weekly cash benefit. As Mrs Cole said, 'It is impossible to look after these children properly if there is a constant anxiety about money.'

Notes and references

Introduction

1 S. Baldwin, 'The financial consequences of disablement in children', D. Phil. thesis, University of York, Department of Social Policy and Social Work, 1982, 2 vols.

Chapter 1 Financial provision for disablement in children

1 *Social Security Provision for Chronically Sick and Disabled People*, HC 276, London, HMSO, 1974. The review had come about because, during the final stages of the Social Security Bill 1973, MPs expressed strong dissatisfaction with existing provision. A clause was therefore inserted in the 1973 Social Security Act (Section 36) requiring the Secretary of State to review provision and report to Parliament by 31 October 1974.
2 Ibid., para. 45.
3 Ibid., Introduction, para. 6 and para. 45 of the text.
4 B. Abel-Smith and P. Townsend, *The Poor and the Poorest*, Occasional Papers on Social Administration, London, Bell, 1965; S. Sainsbury, *Registered as Disabled*, Occasional Papers on Social Administration, London, Bell, 1970; A. I. Harris, E. Cox and C. R. W. Smith, *Handicapped and Impaired in Great Britain*, London, HMSO, 1971.
5 For a discussion of the Chronically Sick and Disabled Persons Act and its passage through Parliament see W. Jaehnig, 'Seeking out the disabled', in K. Jones (ed.), *The Year Book of Social Policy in Britain 1972*, London, Routledge & Kegan Paul, 1973.
6 T. Lynes, 'Creating a national disability income', *New Society*, vol. 24, pp. 244–6.
7 For example, a review of European provision for disablement – 'Cash benefits for the handicapped; a selective study of the schemes of some European countries', DHSS, unpublished.
8 Earnings-relation in benefits for unemployment, sickness and industrial injuries was introduced in the National Insurance Act of 1966; the Chronically Sick and Disabled Persons Act was enacted in 1970; the attendance allowance was introduced in the National Insurance Act 1970; invalidity benefit was introduced in the National Insurance Act 1971 (para. 3); non-contributory invalidity pension was introduced in the Social Security Act 1975.
9 Section 36, Social Security Act 1973, c. 38.
10 *National Superannuation and Social Insurance*, Cmnd 3883, London, HMSO, 1969.

11 National Insurance Act 1970, Section 4, c. 51.
12 Pages 95–6 and 97–9.
13 Harris *et al.*, op. cit.
14 J. Bradshaw, *The Family Fund: An Initiative in Social Policy*, London, Routledge & Kegan Paul, 1980, pp. 19–32.
15 Sir Keith Joseph, for example, in the course of the debate during which the establishment of the Family Fund was announced, referred to the services already being provided 'by statutory and voluntary services to the families concerned' as though these were providing most of the help families needed (*House of Commons Debates*, vol. 847, col. 446).
16 It is probable that children's needs were assumed not to be sufficiently different from those of disabled adults to justify the extra cost of extending the survey to include a representative sample of disabled children.
17 HC 276, op. cit., para. 6.
18 For example, G. Myrdal, *Beyond the Welfare State*, London, Duckworth, 1960.
19 P. Hall, H. Land, R. Parker and A. Webb, *Change, Choice and Conflict in Social Policy*, London, Heinemann, 1975.
20 Bradshaw, op. cit., p. 7.
21 H. Sjöström and R. Nilsson, *Thalidomide and the Power of the Drug Companies*, Harmondsworth, Middx, Penguin Books, 1972; the *Sunday Times*, *The Thalidomide Children and the Law*, London, André Deutsch, 1973; D. Mason, *Thalidomide, My Fight*, London, Allen & Unwin, 1976.
22 Bradshaw, op. cit., p. 7.
23 E. Younghusband, D. Birchall, R. Davie and M. L. Kellmer Pringle (eds), *Living with Handicap*, London, National Children's Bureau, 1970.
24 *House of Commons Debates*, vol. 847, col. 446, 1972.
25 Ibid.
26 Royal Commission on Civil Liability and Compensation for Personal Injury, Chairman: Lord Pearson, *Report*, Cmnd 7054, London, HMSO, 1978.
27 For example, the 1974 debate on vaccine-damaged children, *House of Commons Debate*, vol. 882, cols 1514–26, and the eventual legislation, Vaccine Damage Payments Acts, c. 17.
28 Congenital Disabilities (Civil Liability) Act 1976.
29 Report of the Committee on Child Health Services, Chairman: Professor D. Court, *Fit for the Future*, Cmnd 6684, London, HMSO, 1976; Report of the Committee of Enquiry into the Education of Handicapped Children and Young People, Chairman: M. Warnock, *Special Educational Needs*, Cmnd 7212, London, HMSO, 1978.
30 For example, F. S. W. Brimblecombe, 'An Exeter project for handicapped children', *British Medical Journal*, IV, 706, 1974; A. Shearer, *A Community Service for Mentally Handicapped Children – Barnardo's Chorley Project*, London, Barnardo Social Work Paper No. 4, 1978.

31 For a discussion of the issues involved, see: Anon., 'Ethical problems in the management of some severely handicapped children', *Journal of Medical Ethics*, September 1981, pp. 117–24; J. Finch, 'The Arthur judgment', *Nursing Mirror*, vol. 153, no. 21, pp. 12–13; I. Kennedy, 'Reflections on the Arthur trial', *New Society*, 7 January 1982, pp. 13–15; Glanville Williams, 'Down's syndrome and the duty to preserve life', *New Law Journal*, 8 October 1981, pp. 1040–1.
32 P. S. Atiyah, *Accidents, Compensation and the Law*, London, Weidenfeld & Nicolson, 1970; T. Ison, *The Forensic Lottery*, St Albans, Herts, Staples Press, 1967.
33 Royal Commission of Inquiry, *Report on Compensation for Personal Injury in New Zealand*, December 1972 (The Woodhouse Report), New Zealand, Government Printer, 1972.
34 Atiyah, op. cit., p. 603.
35 The inadequacies of the tort system were highlighted by a survey conducted by the Centre for Socio-legal Studies, Wolfson College, Oxford University. The results of that survey are reported in D. R. Harris et al., *Compensation and Support for Illness and Injury*, London, Macmillan (forthcoming).
36 A. Walker and P. Townsend, 'Compensation for disability: the wrong course', in M. Brown and S. Baldwin (eds), *The Year Book of Social Policy in Britain 1978*, London, Routledge & Kegan Paul, 1979.
37 *Safety and Health at Work*, Report of the Committee 1970–2, Chairman: Lord Robens, Cmnd 5034, London, HMSO, 1972, p. 149.
38 *Hansard*, 19 December 1972, para. 1120.
39 For example, Walker and Townsend, op. cit.; A. Ogus, P. Corfield and D. R. Harris, 'Pearson: principled reform or political compromise?', Centre for Socio-legal Studies, Wolfson College, Oxford University, 1978 (mimeographed typescript).
40 Pearson Report, op. cit., ch. 4, para. 45.
41 A. Walker and M. Maclean, 'Financial compensation for personal injury: a case-study in law and social policy', unpublished paper given at a seminar on tort and its alternatives at the Centre for Socio-legal Studies, Wolfson College, Oxford University on 28 March 1980.
42 Ibid.
43 Atiyah, op. cit., p. 449.
44 G. Williams and B. A. Hepple, *Foundations of the Law of Tort*, London, Butterworths, 1976; R. F. C. Henston (ed.), *Salmond on the Law of Torts*, 17th edn, London, Sweet & Maxwell, 1977.
45 Atiyah, op. cit.; Ison, op. cit.
46 Pearson Report, op. cit.
47 Atiyah, op. cit., pp. 521–7.
48 Pearson Report, op. cit., para. 339.
49 Ibid., para. 351.
50 Ibid., para. 360.
51 Ibid., para. 363.
52 Atiyah, op. cit., p. 341.
53 An income as of right was not available for non-industrially-disabled

people till 1975. The Social Security Act of that year introduced the new non-contributory invalidity pension (NCIP) proposed in the 1974 White Paper. Ironically, however, NCIP was set at only 60 per cent of the contributory invalidity pension and many disabled people remained dependent, therefore, on means-tested supplementary benefit.
54 The only exception to this is where unemployment benefit is lost for 6 weeks when employment has been left 'without just cause'.
55 Walker and Maclean, op. cit., p. 10.
56 L. D. McClements, *The Economics of Social Security*, London, Heinemann, 1978, p. 32.
57 R. M. Titmuss, 'Welfare state and welfare society', in R. M. Titmuss, *Commitment to Welfare*, London, Allen & Unwin, 1968, pp. 131–3.
58 P. Jones, 'Rights, welfare and stigma', in N. Timms (ed.), *Social Welfare: Why and How?*, London, Routledge & Kegan Paul, 1980, p. 125.
59 McClements, op. cit., p. 32.
60 Pearson Report, op. cit., paras 27–8.
61 Ibid., para. 29.
62 Ibid., para. 1488.
63 Children were treated, therefore, as critics of Pearson would have preferred all disabled people to be – i.e. that social security provision should ignore the origins of the disablement and focus only on its severity. The exception was vaccine-damaged children for whom special provision was recommended and subsequently introduced.
64 See J. Bradshaw and D. Lawton, 'An examination of equity in the administration of the attendance allowance', *Policy and Politics*, vol. 8, no. 1, 39–54; K. R. Cooke, 'An evaluation of the mobility allowance for families with handicapped children', *Child: Care, Health and Development*, 6, 1980, pp. 279–89.
65 J. Finch and D. Groves, 'Community care and the family: a case for equal opportunities?', *Journal of Social Policy*, vol. 9, part 4, pp. 487–511.
66 For example, E. Topliss, *Provision for the Disabled*, London, Basil Blackwell and Martin Robertson, 1975.
67 J. Tizard and J. C. Grad, *The Mentally Handicapped and their Families*, Oxford, Oxford University Press, 1961; S. Hewett, *The Family and the Handicapped Child*, London, Allen & Unwin, 1970; E. Younghusband *et al.*, op. cit.
68 *House of Commons Debates*, op. cit; HC 276, op. cit.
69 The work of the Family Fund Research Team is summarized in Bradshaw, 1980, op. cit. An example of other work is the research on disabled children carried out under the direction of Professor Neville Butler at the University of Bristol. For example, N. Butler, R. Gill, D. Pomeroy and J. Fewtrell, 'The handicapped child at home', *Residential Social Work*, vol. 17, no. 8, 1977, pp. 225–8.
70 Pearson Report, op. cit., paras 1507–8.
71 Bradshaw, 1980, op. cit., pp. 205–7.
72 Pearson Report, op. cit., para. 1521.
73 Ibid.

Chapter 2 Disabled children – rights to compensation?

1 See, for example, J. Carrier and I. Kendall, 'The development of welfare states', in *Journal of Social Policy*, vol. 6, 3, 1973, pp. 271–90; R. Mishra, *Society and Social Policy: Theoretical Perspectives on State Welfare*, London, Macmillan, 1973; D. Miller, *Social Justice*, Oxford, Clarendon Press, 1976; R. Nozick, *Anarchy, State and Utopia*, Oxford, Blackwell, 1974; R. Plant, H. Lesser, P. Taylor-Gooby, *Political Philosophy and Social Welfare*, London, Routledge & Kegan Paul, 1980; N. Timms (ed.), *Social Welfare: Why and How?*, London, Routledge & Kegan Paul, 1980; A. Weale, *Political Theory and Social Policy*, London, Routledge & Kegan Paul, 1983.
2 Throughout this chapter the terms 'state', 'society' and 'community' are used interchangeably, though they are not identical concepts. They are used interchangeably because for the purposes of this discussion the state is viewed as the agency through which the obligations of individuals living in society are discharged.
3 R. Plant, 'The moral basis of welfare provision', in Plant, Lesser and Taylor-Gooby, op. cit., p. 52.
4 R. M. Titmuss, *The Gift Relationship*, Harmondsworth, Middx, Penguin Books, 1970, pp. 212 et passim.
5 R. Plant, 'Markets, community and welfare', in Plant, Lesser and Taylor-Gooby, op. cit., p. 243.
6 R. Plant, in Plant, Lesser and Taylor-Gooby, op. cit., pp. 52–3.
7 R. M. Titmuss, *Social Policy*, London, Allen & Unwin, 1974, p. 141.
8 A. Walker, 'Justice and disability', in K. Jones and S. Baldwin (eds), *The Year Book of Social Policy in Britain 1975*, London, Routledge & Kegan Paul, 1976, pp. 192–212.
9 W. B. Gallie, 'Essentially contested concepts', *Proceedings of the Aristotelian Society*, 1955–56, London, Harrison & Son, 1956, pp. 167–98.
10 The most notable attempt to do so in recent years has been that of J. Rawls (*A Theory of Justice*, Oxford, Clarendon Press, 1972). For an account of weaknesses in Rawls's argument, see Miller, op. cit.
11 The most original and best developed statement of this position can be found in Miller, op. cit.
12 J. Bradshaw, 'A taxonomy of social need', in G. McLachlan (ed.), *Problems and Progress in Medical Care*, Oxford, Oxford University Press, 1972, pp. 69–82; A. Forder, *Concepts in Social Administration*, London, Routledge & Kegan Paul, 1974, p. 39; Plant, Lesser and Taylor-Gooby, op. cit., pp. 20–36.
13 See, for example, D. Nevitt, 'Demand and need', in H. Heisler (ed.), *Foundations of Social Administration*, London, Macmillan, 1977, pp. 125–6; A. Williams, 'Need as a demand concept', in A. Culyer (ed.), *Economic Policies and Social Goals*, Oxford, Martin Robertson, 1974, pp. 60–76.
14 P. Jones, 'Rights, welfare and stigma', in Timms (ed.), op. cit., pp. 130–6.
15 Plant, Lesser and Taylor-Gooby, op. cit., p. 28.

16 For a full statement of this argument see P. Jones, 'Rights, welfare and stigma', in Timms (ed.), op. cit.
17 For example, H. B. Acton, *The Morals of Markets*, London, Longman, 1971; Sir N. Anderson, *Liberty, Law and Justice* (Hamlyn Lectures, 30th series), London, Stevens, 1978, pp. 43–4; M. Cranston, *What Are Human Rights?*, London, Bodley Head, 1973; R. Dworkin, *Taking Rights Seriously*, London, Duckworth, 1977; Nozick, op. cit.; D. Raphael (ed.), *Political Theory and the Rights of Man*, London, Macmillan, 1978; Weale, op. cit.
18 R. M. Titmuss, 'Welfare state and welfare society', in R. M. Titmuss, *Commitment to Welfare*, London, Allen & Unwin, 1968, pp. 131–3.
19 P. Jones, 'Rights, welfare and stigma', in Timms (ed.), op. cit., pp. 123–4.
20 In, for example, *The Gift Relationship*, op. cit. and 'Welfare rights, law and discretion', *Political Quarterly*, 1961, p. 116.
21 See, for example, Miller, op. cit.; P. Pettit, *Judging Justice*, London, Routledge & Kegan Paul, 1980, pp. 78–83.
22 P. Jones, 'Rights, welfare and stigma', in Timms (ed.), op. cit., p. 125.
23 For the literature discussing these cases and the issues involved see Chapter 1, note 31.
24 R. M. Moroney, *The Family and the State: Considerations for Social Policy*, London, Longman, 1976, p. 128.
25 H. Land and R. Parker, 'United Kingdom', in S. B. Kamerman and A. J. Kahn (eds), *Family Policy: Government and Families in Fourteen Countries*, New York, Columbia University Press, 1978, pp. 330–66.
26 France, as a country with a highly developed family policy, provides an example of how provision for disablement in children, including good preventive ante-natal services and good social security provision, appears to bear a strong relation to provision for children generally.
27 See, for example, J. Donzelot, *The Policing of Families: Welfare versus the State*, London, Hutchinson, 1979; C. Lasch, *Haven in a Heartless World: the Family Besieged*, New York, Basic Books, 1978.
28 F. Engels, *The Origin of the Family, Private Property and the State*, London, Lawrence & Wishart, 1972; J. S. Mill, 'The subjection of women', in R. Fletcher (ed.), *John Stuart Mill: A Logical Critique of Sociology*, Sunbury-on-Thames, Nelson, 1973, pp. 349–61.
29 The conflict between women's rights and community care policies is examined in J. Finch and D. Groves, 'Community care and the family: a case for equal opportunities?', *Journal of Social Policy*, vol. 9, part 4, pp. 487 511.
30 Moroney, op. cit., p. 27.
31 J. Bowlby, *Maternal Care and Mental Health*, Geneva, World Health Organisation, 1951.
32 For example, E. Goffman, *Asylums*, Harmondsworth, Middx, Penguin Books, 1961; *Stigma*, New Jersey, Prentice-Hall, 1963; M. Oswin, *The Empty Hours*, London, Allen Lane, 1971; J. Tizard, R.

D. King, N. V. Raynes and W. Yule, 'The care and treatment of subnormal children in institutions', paper presented at the International Conference of the Association of Special Education, London, 1966.

33 It is possible to present a similar argument, not in relation to the distribution of burdens in society, but to the distribution of welfare. It could be argued that a powerful value in highly developed countries is that goods ought not to be distributed so that some people are left with an unreasonable share. The effect of disablement in a child may be to leave families with an inequitable share of welfare because of income losses and extra costs. If this does happen then a weak principle of equitable distribution would, Weale (personal communication) argues, dictate that families with disabled children ought to receive more income than families in similar circumstances without disabled children. They ought, similarly, to receive a higher volume of services or the means of obtaining these to compensate for their inequitable share of leisure.

34 p. 22.

35 A. C. Pigou, *The Economics of Welfare*, London, Macmillan, 1920.

36 R. M. Titmuss, 'Social costs and social change', in Titmuss, 1974, op. cit., p. 60.

37 Ibid., p. 74.

38 J. Kleinig, 'Human rights, legal rights and social change', in E. Kamanka and A. E. Tay (eds), *Human Rights*, London, Arnold, 1978, pp. 36–47.

Chapter 3   Measuring the costs of disablement

1 See, for example, G. S. Becker, 'A theory of the allocation of time', *Economic Journal*, vol. LXXV, no. 299, 1965, pp. 493–517; R. Gronau, 'The effect of children on the housewife's value of time', *Journal of Political Economy*, vol. 81, 1973, pp. S168–99; R. A. Pollack and M. L. Wachter, 'The relevance of the household production function and its implications for the allocation of time', *Journal of Political Economy*, vol. 83, 1975, pp. 255–77.

2 These adjustments are discussed in relation to households with an adult disabled member in Y. Brittan and I. G. Vlachonikolis, 'The effect of ill-health and subsequent compensation and support on household income', Centre for Socio-legal Studies, Wolfson College, Oxford University, Working Paper No. 6, July 1980.

3 For a discussion of the problems involved in comparing living standards from income and expenditure data and a review of the literature on this subject see P. Townsend, *Poverty in the United Kingdom*, Harmondsworth, Middx, Penguin Books, 1979, pp. 262–7. For a review of the literature on the cost of children see J. van der Gaag, 'On measuring the cost of children', University of Wisconsin, Madison, Institute for Research on Poverty, Discussion Paper, 1981.

4 B. Abel-Smith and P. Townsend, *The Poor and the Poorest*, Occasional Papers on Social Administration, London, Bell, 1965.

5 A. I. Harris, E. Cox and C. R. W. Smith, *Handicapped and Impaired in Great Britain*, Part III, Incomes and Entitlement to Supplementary Benefit of Impaired People in Great Britain, London, HMSO, 1972.
6 Townsend, op. cit.
7 R. Layard, D. Piachaud and M. Stewart, Royal Commission on the Distribution of Income and Wealth, Report No. 6, *Lower Incomes*, London, HMSO, 1978, pp. 107–13.
8 For example, S. Sainsbury, *Registered as Disabled*, Occasional Papers on Social Administration, London, Bell, 1970; M. Hyman, *The Extra Costs of Disabled Living*, London, National Fund for Research into Crippling Diseases and Disablement Income Group, 1977; Disability Alliance, Pamphlet series on disablement; R. Stowell, *Disabled People on Supplementary Benefit*, London, Disablement Income Group, 1980.
9 B. L. Wolfe, 'Impacts of disability and some policy implications; earnings lost and income gained; the equity and adequacy of transfers to the disabled', University of Wisconsin, Madison, Institute for Research on Poverty, Discussion Paper, 1979–80.
10 D. R. Harris *et al.*, *Compensation and Support for Illness and Injury*, London, Macmillan (forthcoming).
11 Sainsbury, op. cit.; M. Blaxter, *The Meaning of Disability*, London, Heinemann, 1976.
12 For a review and bibliography of such studies see L. Durward, *That's the Way the Money Goes: The Extra Cost of Living with a Disability*, Disability Alliance, 1981.
13 A. I. Harris, *et al.*, op. cit.
14 For example, J. Bradshaw, *The Financial Needs of Disabled Children*, Pamphlet No. 2, London, Disability Alliance, 1975; D. Pomeroy *et al.*, *Handicapped Children: Their Homes and Life-styles*, London Department of the Environment, 1978.
15 D. Piachaud, J. Bradshaw and J. Weale, 'The income effect of a disabled child', *Journal of Epidemiology and Community Health*, vol. 35, no. 2, June 1981, pp. 123–7.
16 See, for example, S. Baldwin, 'Families with handicapped children', in K. Jones and S. Baldwin (eds), *The Year Book of Social Policy in Britain 1975*, London, Routledge & Kegan Paul, 1976, pp. 171–91; S. Baldwin, *Disabled Children – Counting the Costs*, Pamphlet No. 8, London, Disability Alliance, 1977; J. Bradshaw (1975), op. cit.; L. Burton, *The Family Life of Sick Children*, London, Routledge & Kegan Paul, 1975; Townsend, op. cit., pp. 745–52; M. F. Woodburn, *Social Implications of Spina Bifida*, London, ASBAH, 1973.
17 See, for example, N. Butler, R. Gill, D. Pomeroy and J. Fewtrell, 'The handicapped child at home', *Residential Social Work*, vol. 17, no. 8, 1977, pp. 225–8.
18 For a review of this work see J. Bradshaw, *The Family Fund: An Initiative in Social Policy*, London, Routledge & Kegan Paul, 1980.
19 C. M. Bodkin *et al.*, 'Financial burdens of childhood cancer', *British Medical Journal*, 1982, 284, pp. 1542–4; S. Kew, 'The cost of handicap', *British Hospital Journal*, vol. LXXXIII, no. 4330, 1973.

20 Baldwin (1976), op. cit.
21 Baldwin (1977), op. cit.
22 Hyman, op. cit.
23 It was restricted to people living in one London borough.
24 W. F. F. Kemsley, 'Collecting data on economic flow variables using interviews and record-keeping', in L. Moss and H. Goldstein (eds), *The Recall Method in Social Surveys*, University of London, Institute of Education, 1979, p. 127; Kemsley, Redpath and Holmes, op. cit., chapter 14.

Chapter 4 The study – design and methods

1 The Family Fund register contains a higher proportion of manual heads of household than the population at large. This may reflect the Fund's purpose of helping families in need. It may, on the other hand, reflect the incidence of severe disablement. Recent analysis of a ten-year-old cohort of disabled children suggests that there may be a higher incidence of disablement in children in the lower social classes. See '1970 cohort 10 year follow-up study. Interim report', DHSS 108/6.82.KC. (Unpublished report by the Social Policy Research Unit, University of York.)
2 W. F. F. Kemsley, R. U. Redpath, M. Holmes, *Family Expenditure Survey Handbook*, London, HMSO, 1980.
3 The expenditure diaries used in the FES do not require respondents to record for which member of the family purchases are made. This means that it is almost impossible to identify the extent to which the disabled child's extra expenses are met by spending less on other family members. Purchases of meat, for example, may include more expensive high-protein cuts, bought for the disabled child, and cheaper cuts bought for others in the family. An additional problem is that the FES coding frame makes it difficult to isolate expenditure necessitated by particular aspects of disability. Expenditure caused by incontinence, for example, occurs under a number of headings – toiletries, infants' clothing, children's clothing, cleaning materials, etc. These categories contain general family spending as well as special expenditure necessitated by the child's incontinence.
4 The latest FES data available at the time of the study was for the 1975 survey. The characteristics of respondents to the 1975 FES who met the criteria for this study were used to predict the characteristics of similar families taking part in the FES in 1978.
5 The General Index of Retail Prices, for example, rose by only 4.1 per cent over the whole period of the study.
6 Office of Population Censuses and Surveys, *Classification of Occupations, 1970*, London, HMSO, 1970.
7 Notes of guidance as to what constitutes very severe disability according to the Family Fund's criteria can be found in the Fund's handbook – *The Family Fund and How it Helps* – which is available from the Fund's headquarters in York.
8 For discussion of the description and classification of disablement see

D. Duckworth, *The Classification and Measurement of Disablement*, London, HMSO, 1983; P. H. N. Wood, *Classification of Impairments and Handicaps*, Geneva, World Health Organisation, 1975. The terms 'impairment' and 'disability' are used interchangeably throughout this book to represent the effect of a disease or disorder on certain organs or the way this affects bodily functions that are important in daily living such as mobility, speech or continence. This is distinguished from 'handicap' – the dependency created by disabilities or impairments. In general children are referred to as disabled rather than handicapped except where the term 'handicapped' is used in the source quoted.

9 Here, as throughout the book, children's names have been altered to preserve confidentiality.

10 For example, J. Copeland (ed.), *For the Love of Ann*, London, Arrow, 1973; A. Gath, *Down's Syndrome and the Family*, London, Academic Press, 1978; C. Glendinning, *Unshared Care? Parents and their Disabled Children*, London, Routledge & Kegan Paul, 1983; S. Gregory, *The Deaf Child and his Family*, London, Allen & Unwin, 1976; C. Hannam, *Parents and Mentally Handicapped Children*, Harmondsworth, Middx, Penguin Books, 1975; S. Hewett, *The Family and the Handicapped Child*, London, Allen & Unwin, 1970; J. McMichael, *Handicap*, St Albans, Herts, Staples Press, 1971; M. Voysey, *A Constant Burden*, London, Routledge & Kegan Paul, 1975; J. Wilks and E. Wilks, *Bernard: Bringing up our Mongol Son*, London, Routledge & Kegan Paul, 1974.

Chapter 5 Incomes

1 The income concepts used in this study were those of the FES. FES questions were used throughout in collecting information on income and FES procedures replicated in creating different income definitions. Detailed information on these definitions can be found in the FES handbook by W. F. F. Kemsley, R. U. Redpath and M. Holmes, *Family Expenditure Survey Handbook*, London, HMSO, 1980, in the FES reports which are published annually by HMSO and in the Department of Employment's FES Users Information Pack. Briefly the basic income concept used in the FES is that of gross weekly cash income from all sources at the time of the interview. This includes all earnings, pensions and income from annuities, social security benefits and other benefits and allowances, income from investments and property and other non-earned income. Where families are living in owner-occupied or rent-free accommodation a weekly imputed income is added to their other income to represent the gain arising from the absence of housing costs. This imputed income is based on the dwelling's rateable value.

2 See, for example, Central Policy Review Staff, *Services for Young Children with Working Mothers*, London, HMSO, 1978; Department of Employment, *Women and Work: A Review* (Manpower [sic] Paper No. 11), London, HMSO, 1978; Department of Employment,

Annual Report 1978–9, London, HMSO, 1979; Equal Opportunities Commission, *Women and Low Incomes*, November 1977, Manchester, EOC; N. Fonda and P. Moss (eds), *Mothers in Employment*, London, Brunel University and Thomas Coram Research Unit, 1977; L. Hamill, *Wives as Sole and Joint Breadwinners*, Government Economic Working Paper No. 13, London, HMSO, 1978; A. Hunt, *A Survey of Women's Employment, 1965*, London, HMSO, 1968; A. Hunt *et al.*, *Families and their Needs*, London, HMSO, 1973; R. Layard, D. Piachaud and M. Stewart, Royal Commission on the Distribution of Income and Wealth, Report No. 6, *Lower Incomes*, London, HMSO, 1978; M. McNay and C. Pond, *Low Pay and Family Poverty*, Study Commission on the Family Occasional Paper No. 2, London, SCF, 1980; P. Moss and N. Fonda (eds), *Work and the Family*, London, Temple-Smith, 1980; Royal Commission on the Distribution of Income and Wealth, Report No. 6, *Lower Incomes*, Addendum by G. Doughty, D. Lea and D. Wedderburn, London, HMSO, 1978.
3 See, for example, Hamill, op. cit.; Layard *et al.*, op. cit.
4 There is a considerable literature, both British and American, on married women's labour-force participation. For a useful review of this literature see R. Layard, M. Barton and A. Zabalza, 'Married women's participation and hours', *Economica*, 47, 1980, pp. 51–72. The American literature is reviewed in S. Danziger *et al.*, 'How income transfer programs affect work, savings and income distribution: a critical review', *Journal of Economic Literature*, 19 : 3, 1981, pp. 975–1028.
5 Previous research on the employment of women with disabled children is summarized in M. Philp, *Children with Disabilities and their Families: A Review of Research*, Windsor, NFER-Nelson, 1982.
6 For example, N. Butler *et al.*, *Housing Problems of Handicapped People in Bristol*, University of Bristol, Child Health Research Unit, 1976.
7 This table is based on all wives of non-self-employed men. Participating women are defined as those who were employed or self-employed in the survey period. Earnings calculations are based only on those employed women who actually worked and earned in the survey period. Self-employed women are excluded in the calculation of hours worked because FES does not collect detailed information on their hours.
8 R. Layard *et al.*, *The Causes of Poverty*, Background Paper No. 5 to Report No. 6 of the Royal Commission on the Distribution of Income and Wealth, London, HMSO, 1978.
9 J. Hurstfield, *The Part-Time Trap*, London, Low Pay Unit, 1978.
10 C. Glendinning, *Unshared Care? Parents and their Disabled Children*, London, Routledge & Kegan Paul, 1983.
11 This is discussed in P. Moss, 'Parents at work', in Moss and Fonda, op. cit.
12 C. Hakim, *Occupational Segregation*, Department of Employment Research Paper No. 9, November 1979.

13 P. Moss, 'Parents at work', in Moss and Fonda, op. cit.
14 The absence of information on the working lives of men with children is discussed in P. Moss, 'The current situation', in Fonda and Moss, op. cit. The existing literature on the employment of fathers is discussed in P. Moss, 'Parents at work', in Moss and Fonda, op. cit.
15 L. Burton, *The Family Life of Sick Children*, London, Routledge & Kegan Paul, 1975.
16 Information on the earnings of men whose main job was in self-employment was not included in the comparative part of the study. These men's views were, however, included in the section dealing with subjective views of the disabled child's effect on their working lives since there seemed no reason to think this information was unreliable.
17 Differences in the samples' occupation structures and the reasons for these are discussed in Chapter 4 (pp. 66–7) and in Appendix 1.
18 The FES's concern is with normal rather than actual earnings. Where actual earnings in the last pay period are different from normal earnings the normal earnings figure is used.
19 Presumably since women's earnings fall as the severity of the condition increases men with more severely disabled children experience some pressure to increase their own earnings to compensate for the reduction in or absence of earnings by their wives.
20 This is corroborated by Wilkin's study of families with mentally handicapped children – D. Wilkin, *Caring for the Mentally Handicapped Child*, London, Croom Helm, 1979.
21 This was done by reweighting the sample of families with disabled children so that its occupation structure was identical to that of the FES sample. This exercise demonstrated that the differences observed in men's earnings were not mainly due to their different occupation structures but to differences in the earnings of men (with and without disabled children) in similar occupations at the time of the study. Before reweighting the difference in the samples' average weekly earnings had been £8.70; reweighting made a difference of less than £1 a week.
22 K. R. Cooke and F. M. Staden, *The Impact of the Mobility Allowance: An Evaluative Study*, London, HMSO, 1981.
23 Two measures of the overall severity of the child's condition were used. Severity of disability was measured by assessing the severity of each of eleven disabilities (or impairments) as absent, moderate or severe and assigning a score of 0, 1 or 2 as appropriate. These scores were then added up to give each child an overall severity rating. The areas of possible impairment were: mobility, use of hands, sight, hearing, speech, continence, IQ, fits, (hyper)activity, susceptibility to severe pain or trauma. Severity of handicap was measured using a similar procedure for seven possible areas of dependency: in washing, dressing, feeding, moving around independently, toileting, supervision by day and attendance at night.
24 K. R. Cooke, 'An evaluation of the mobility allowance for families with handicapped children', *Child: Care, Health and Development*, 6,

1980, pp. 279–89.
25 Royal Commission on Civil Liability and Compensation for Personal Injury, Chairman: Lord Pearson, *Report*, Cmnd 7054, London, HMSO, 1978, paras 1533–4.
26 See pages 119–200.
27 See, for example, Cooke and Staden, op. cit.
28 This is primarily an income, rather than a social class effect. Non-manual families were almost invariably richer than manual families. However the small group of very poor, non-manual families with disabled children – those with very young children – were better off than their FES counterparts. Income data is presented for non-manual and manual families separately because the proportions of non-manual and manual families in the two samples were different.
29 Since the vast majority of families in both samples would have been ineligible for the long-term rate had they applied for supplementary benefit their disposable incomes are expressed as a proportion of the short-term rate. Housing costs are deducted from disposable income in this calculation because supplementary benefit claimants' housing costs are met.
30 Calculated from actual changes in average earnings up to April 1983 (source: Department of Employment *Gazette*) and predicted increases to April 1984.

Chapter 6 Expenditure

1 For a review of work in this field and an extensive bibliography see M. Philp, *Children with Disabilities and their Families: A Review of Research*, Windsor, NFER-Nelson, 1982, and L. Durward, *That's the Way the Money Goes: The Extra Cost of Living with a Disability*, London, Disability Alliance, 1981. More recently the costs of childhood cancer have been highlighted in C. M. Bodkin *et al.*, 'Financial burdens of childhood cancer', *British Medical Journal*, 1982, 284, pp. 1542–4.
2 There is of course a danger that respondents will either falsify their expenditure or change their behaviour. It is thought that commodities like tobacco and alcohol are particularly susceptible to this kind of 'contamination' by the research. For a discussion of these issues see W. F. F. Kemsley, 'Collecting data on economic flow variables using interviews and record-keeping', in L. Moss and H. Goldstein (eds), *The Recall Method in Social Surveys*, University of London, 1979, p. 127; W. F. F. Kemsley, R. U. Redpath and M. Holmes, *Family Expenditure Survey Handbook*, London, HMSO, 1980, pp. 49–54.
3 Very few families, in a sample of this size, will purchase large items such as cars or washing machines during the survey period. Hence expenditure data for such items is unreliable. As the FES published reports show, standard errors for expenditure on durables is very large.
4 Beyond that a very large number of individual items can be

separately identified from the FES tape.
5 Other goods and miscellaneous goods are treated as separate commodity groups in the FES. Here they have been treated as one commodity group.
6 These are fairly broad income ranges. This was unavoidable if we were to have a sufficient number of observations for analysis, particularly for items such as clothing where purchases are relatively infrequent. Differences in the number of families in the two samples with very high incomes made it necessary to use an income cut-off of £150 so that we would be comparing the expenditure patterns of families with similar incomes.
7 This has been done only for families with disposable incomes between £70 and £100 because of the small numbers in the lowest and highest income ranges.
8 Like all the costs discussed in this chapter, food costs have increased since 1978. It would have been possible, if somewhat tedious, to update expenditure on each item to take account of inflation. (The overall rate of inflation in the period 1978–84 was of the order of 5 per cent per annum, though this varies between commodities.) It was decided however, that adjusting the data to this extent was undesirable since it would mean losing touch completely with what families had actually spent. We chose only to update the figure for the total extra costs borne by the families with disabled children (see pp. 128–32). This creates a more appropriate framework for the discussion of appropriate forms and levels of financial support.
9 For example, S. Baldwin, *Disabled Children – Counting the Costs*, Pamphlet No. 8, London, Disability Alliance, 1977; 'Clothing the very severely handicapped child', FF 6/3.74 J. B. (Unpublished working paper – Social Policy Research Unit Working Paper, University of York.)
10 K. R. Cooke and F. M. Staden, *The Impact of the Mobility Allowance: An Evaluative Study*, London, HMSO, 1981.
11 S. Baldwin, 'Families with handicapped children', in K. Jones and S. Baldwin (eds), *The Year Book of Social Policy in Britain 1975*, London, Routledge & Kegan Paul, 1976, pp. 171–91; S. Baldwin, *Disabled Children – Counting the Costs*, London, Disability Alliance, 1977; M. F. Woodburn, *Social Implications of Spina Bifida*, London, ASBAH, 1973.
12 The housing costs figure used in the FES published reports bears no relation to the actual outgoings of owner-occupiers but is based on the rateable value of the dwelling. This is because, for owner-occupiers, it is virtually impossible to make true comparisons of 'housing costs' from actual outgoings on mortgages and rates. Owner occupiers' mortgage repayments include an element of investment which is difficult to allow for. Mortgage repayments may also be higher or lower than the amount strictly needed to pay off the loan – either because buyers have come to an arrangement to pay more or less or because of links with insurance. The difficulties of comparing housing costs are further exacerbated by regional vari-

ation in house prices. The FES figure represents an attempt to measure the value of owner-occupied housing by assessing, from the rateable value, the rent the house could command. Here, however, it was decided that actual outgoings on mortgages and rates were of more direct relevance. (Housing costs are discussed in detail in Kemsley et al., op. cit).
13 D. Pomeroy, et al., *Handicapped Children: Their Homes and Life-Styles*, London, Department of the Environment, 1978.
14 For a full list of what is included in these and the other main commodity groups see the FES published reports.
15 This analysis is presented in full in S. Baldwin, 'The financial consequences of disablement in children', D. Phil. thesis, University of York, Department of Social Policy and Social Work, 1982, Vol. 1, pp. 338–60.
16 Detailed figures for families in all three income ranges can be found in Baldwin (1982), op. cit.
17 The 1984 figure was obtained by updating the overall difference in the two groups' expenditures to take account of the differences in the General Index of Retail Prices between February 1978 and February 1984. As already noted (ref. 8 above), it was neither desirable nor practicable to do this for each individual item compared.
18 FES expenditure diaries are kept for only fourteen days. Expenditure records for such a short period will not necessarily give a true idea of the family's typical expenditure pattern. One family may, for example, buy a large quantity of food in bulk and also buy the children's clothes for the summer while another family may happen to have done this in the previous week and buy scarcely anything in the diary-keeping period. For this reason it is possible only to analyse the expenditure of groups of families.
19 This investigation, which consisted of examining typical permutations of extra costs, is described in Baldwin (1982), op. cit.
20 For the middle-income families with disabled children average total expenditure was 101 per cent of their average disposable incomes, whereas for the richest families it was 93 per cent. (For the families in the control the respective figures were 95 per cent and 80 per cent.)
21 These costs are discussed in considerably more detail in Baldwin (1982), op. cit.

Chapter 7 The overall effect – ways of coping and expectations of help

1 A. Gray, 'The working class family as an economic unit', in C. Harris (ed.), *The Sociology of the Family*, London, Sociological Review Monograph, 1979; J. Pahl, 'Patterns of money management within marriage', *Journal of Social Policy*, 9, 3, 1980, pp. 313–15.
2 There were three interviewers apart from the author, chosen because they were social workers experienced in working with disabled children and their families or had research experience in the field of budgeting and money management among low-incomes families.
3 See, for example, P. Ashley, *Money, Deprivation and the Poor*,

London, Heinemann, 1983; A. Gray, 'Family budgeting systems', in N. Newman (ed.), *In Cash or in Kind*, Department of Social Administration, University of Edinburgh, 1975.
4 C. Glendinning, *Unshared Share? Parents and their Disabled Children*, London, Routledge & Kegan Paul, 1983; M. Voysey, *A Constant Burden*, London, Routledge & Kegan Paul, 1975.

Chapter 8 Conclusion

1 A second important reason was that our comparative expenditure data related mainly to everyday costs. Larger capital costs and the costs of hospitalization which do probably rise with the severity of the condition, are not accurately reflected in expenditure data based on fourteen days of record-keeping.
2 J. Bradshaw, *The Family Fund: An Initiative in Social Policy*, London, Routledge & Kegan Paul, 1980, pp. 199–204.
3 Royal Commission on Civil Liability and Compensation for Personal Injury, Chairman: Lord Pearson, *Report*, Cmnd 7054, London, HMSO, 1978, paras 1532–4.
4 'The case for lowering the qualifying age for the mobility allowance to two.' (Unpublished working paper, Social Policy Research Unit, University of York.)
5 For a discussion of the elements of such a scheme see: Disablement Income Group, *Realizing a National Disability Income*, London, DIG, 1974; T. Lynes, 'Creating a national disability income', *New Society*, vol. 24, pp. 244–6; Spastics Society, *Pre-Budget Submission to the Rt. Hon. Sir Geoffrey Howe, QC, MP, Chancellor of the Exchequer*, London, Spastics Society, February 1983; P. Townsend, *Poverty and Disability: The Case for a Comprehensive Income Scheme for Disabled People*, London, Disability Alliance, 1975.
6 Pearson Report, op. cit., paras 1521–31.
7 *The Taxation of Husband and Wife*, Cmnd 8093, London, HMSO, 1980; R. Lister, *Social Priorities in Taxation: A Response to the Green Paper on the Taxation of Husband and Wife*, London, Child Poverty Action Group, 1981.
8 This benefit, which is to replace non-contributory invalidity pension (NCIP) and housewives' non-contributory invalidity pension (HNCIP) is to be introduced in November 1985. It is proposed to restrict eligibility to people whose incapacity is assessed at 80 per cent or more, according to the system of assessment currently used in the Industrial Injuries Scheme.

Index

Abel-Smith, B., 5, 53
achondroplasia, see dwarfism
alcohol costs, 108, 122–3, 129, 145
Alexandra, case of, 38–9
alimentary tract, congenital defects of, 109, 183
All-Party Committee on Disability, 5
altruism, 33–4
arthrogryphosis, 183
Atiyah, P. S., 14, 17, 19–20, 25
attendance allowance, 7, 24, 27–8, 95–9, 101, 102, 106, 114, 137, 139, 141, 154, 157, 162, 163–4, 169, 171, 185
autism, 183

behaviour problems, 70, 77, 82, 84, 109, 110, 115, 117, 118, 134, 142, 143, 148, 153–4, 163, 164, 169
benefits, see attendance allowance; cash benefits for disabled children; compensatory benefit; earnings-replacement benefit; expenses allowance; invalid care allowance; mobility allowance; supplementary benefit
Beveridge Report (1942), 20
bills, deferred payment of, 148, 149
bladder, congenital defects of, 90, 183
Blaxter, M., 54
blindness, 12, 46–7, 146, 183
blood diseases, 183
Bodkin, C. M., 55
bone diseases (excluding brittle bones), 183
Bowlby, J., 45
Bradshaw, J., 7, 9, 30, 35, 168
brittle bones, 79, 183
budgeting patterns and skills, 137, 143–50, 165–6
Burton, L., 55
Butler, N., 55

cancer, childhood, 55, 135, 183
carpets, expenditure on, 124, 134
cars, expenditure on, see transport costs

cash benefits for disabled children: improvements in, 56, 61, 166–74; parents' views of, 154–64, 167, 168; see also attendance allowance; mobility allowance
central nervous system, diseases of (excluding spina bifida), 183
cerebral palsy, 55, 69, 78, 79, 82, 121, 145, 149, 151, 162, 183, 184
charity, 33–4, 37
child-care arrangements, problems in making suitable, 77–9, 80, 85
Child Poverty Action Group, 6
Chronically Sick and Disabled Persons Act (1970), 5
cleaning materials, expenditure on, 109, 127
clothing and footwear costs, 107, 108, 115–17, 128, 129, 130, 186–7
community care, 3, 33, 41
compassion, 32, 33–4
compensation, 13–31; rights to, 32–48
compensatory benefit, 171, 173
congenital abnormalities (excluding Thalidomide), 69, 183
Congenital Disabilities (Civil Liability) Act (1976), 26
consumer durables, expenditure on, 107, 108, 124–5, 129, 131, 132, 133–4, 139, 170; see also under specific commodities
coping strategies, 51–2, 59, 141–50
costs, see expenditure and under specific commodities and services
credit buying, 144, 148
cretinism, 183
Crossman, R. H. S., 7
cystic fibrosis, 55, 69, 84, 109, 111, 149, 152, 183

deafness, 12, 68, 88, 146, 152, 183
debt, 84, 136–9
Department of Employment (DE), 24, 65
Department of Health and Social

207

Security (DHSS), 1, 6–8, 10, 12, 24, 53, 168, 175, 176
diabetes, 109
diet, problems relating to, 109–12, 149
Disability Alliance, 53
Disablement Income Group (DIG), 6, 53
diseases and disorders, 182–3; *see also under specific disorders*
Distillers Company (Biochemicals) Ltd, 9–11
division of labour in the family, 87, 93–4
Down's syndrome, 38, 82, 89, 146, 153, 158, 159, 162, 183
dryers, expenditure on, 112, 114, 115, 134
Du Boisson, M., 6
durable household goods, *see* consumer durables
Durkeim, E., 35
dwarfism (achondroplasia), 183

earnings, 72–94; loss of, 18, 23, 28, 49, 50, 54, 55, 56, 57, 73, 75–7, 82–3, 86, 88, 90–4, 95–6, 103–5, 135, 136, 138, 141, 155, 156, 164, 166, 170, 171, 172–3, 186; mens, 55, 66, 73, 85–94; women's, 55, 73–85
earnings-replacement benefit, 171, 172
employers, attitude of, 83, 87–8, 94
employment patterns of men, 85–94, 105–6; hours of work, 86, 87, 90–4, 141, 172; job changes, 86, 87, 105; job losses, 86, 87–8, 89–90; loss of promotion, 86, 88–9, 94, 105, 141, 185; overtime work, 87, 93; participation rates, 89–91; time off work, 87, 88, 94
employment patterns of women, 55, 73–85, 105; evening work, 81; hours of work, 75–7, 79, 81–4, 105; participation rates, 75; part-time work, 76–7, 81–3, 172; time off work, 77, 81, 82
Engels, F., 43
entertainment, expenditure on, 124, 125, 130, 145
epilepsy, 70, 90, 183
equipment, special, 132, 133, 189
expenditure, 51–63, 67, 107–40, 165, 166; overall, 128–32; *see also under specific commodities and services*
expenses allowance, 30, 171–2

Family Expenditure Survey (FES), 53, 61–8, 107–9, 176–82
Family Fund, 9–12, 24, 26, 27, 30, 55–6, 61–8, 114, 134, 167, 168, 170, 176–83
Family Fund Research Team, 26, 29, 55, 85, 182
family/state responsibilities, 40–5, 167
fares, *see* transport costs
food costs, 107, 108, 109–12, 128, 129, 130
footwear, expenditure on, *see* clothing and footwear costs
freezers, expenditure on, 124, 133
fuel costs, 107, 108, 112–15, 129, 130, 187
furniture, expenditure on, 124, 133, 134, 153–4, 189

General Household Survey (GHS), 53, 55
Goffman, E., 45

haemophilia, 183
Hall, P., 8, 9
Harris, A. I., 5, 7–8, 54
head injuries, 183
hearing, impaired, *see* deafness
heart disease, 82, 89, 120–1, 151, 183
heating costs, *see* fuel costs
Hewett, S., 55
hire purchase, *see* credit buying
Hodgkins disease, 183
holidays, 145, 146, 155
home-ownership, constraints on, 126, 151
hospital: costs associated with in-patient stays, 55, 107, 108, 132, 135–9, 156, 170, 190; costs associated with out-patient appointments, 135
housing costs (including adaptations), 87, 90, 107, 108, 126, 129, 132–3, 139, 149, 166, 170, 188–9
hydrocephalus, 183; *see also* spina bifida
Hyman, M., 56–7
hyperactivity, *see* behaviour problems

income, 53–9, 61–2, 66, 71–106, 165, 166; disposable, 101–4; from social security, 72, 94–106; gross, 71–101; relative to need, 102–3; sources of, 72
incontinence, 70, 81, 84, 114, 115, 117, 124, 131, 133, 134, 142, 143, 161, 184, 186–7

Index

Abel-Smith, B., 5, 53
achondroplasia, *see* dwarfism
alcohol costs, 108, 122–3, 129, 145
Alexandra, case of, 38–9
alimentary tract, congenital defects of, 109, 183
All-Party Committee on Disability, 5
altruism, 33–4
arthrogryphosis, 183
Atiyah, P. S., 14, 17, 19–20, 25
attendance allowance, 7, 24, 27–8, 95–9, 101, 102, 106, 114, 137, 139, 141, 154, 157, 162, 163–4, 169, 171, 185
autism, 183

behaviour problems, 70, 77, 82, 84, 109, 110, 115, 117, 118, 134, 142, 143, 148, 153–4, 163, 164, 169
benefits, *see* attendance allowance; cash benefits for disabled children; compensatory benefit; earnings-replacement benefit; expenses allowance; invalid care allowance; mobility allowance; supplementary benefit
Beveridge Report (1942), 20
bills, deferred payment of, 148, 149
bladder, congenital defects of, 90, 183
Blaxter, M., 54
blindness, 12, 46–7, 146, 183
blood diseases, 183
Bodkin, C. M., 55
bone diseases (excluding brittle bones), 183
Bowlby, J., 45
Bradshaw, J., 7, 9, 30, 35, 168
brittle bones, 79, 183
budgeting patterns and skills, 137, 143–50, 165–6
Burton, L., 55
Butler, N., 55

cancer, childhood, 55, 135, 183
carpets, expenditure on, 124, 134
cars, expenditure on, *see* transport costs

cash benefits for disabled children: improvements in, 56, 61, 166–74; parents' views of, 154–64, 167, 168; *see also* attendance allowance; mobility allowance
central nervous system, diseases of (excluding spina bifida), 183
cerebral palsy, 55, 69, 78, 79, 82, 121, 145, 149, 151, 162, 183, 184
charity, 33–4, 37
child-care arrangements, problems in making suitable, 77–9, 80, 85
Child Poverty Action Group, 6
Chronically Sick and Disabled Persons Act (1970), 5
cleaning materials, expenditure on, 109, 127
clothing and footwear costs, 107, 108, 115–17, 128, 129, 130, 186–7
community care, 3, 33, 41
compassion, 32, 33–4
compensation, 13–31; rights to, 32–48
compensatory benefit, 171, 173
congenital abnormalities (excluding Thalidomide), 69, 183
Congenital Disabilities (Civil Liability) Act (1976), 26
consumer durables, expenditure on, 107, 108, 124–5, 129, 131, 132, 133–4, 139, 170; *see also under specific commodities*
coping strategies, 51–2, 59, 141–50
costs, *see* expenditure *and under specific commodities and services*
credit buying, 144, 148
cretinism, 183
Crossman, R. H. S., 7
cystic fibrosis, 55, 69, 84, 109, 111, 149, 152, 183

deafness, 12, 68, 88, 146, 152, 183
debt, 84, 136–9
Department of Employment (DE), 24, 65
Department of Health and Social

207

Security (DHSS), 1, 6–8, 10, 12, 24, 53, 168, 175, 176
diabetes, 109
diet, problems relating to, 109–12, 149
Disability Alliance, 53
Disablement Income Group (DIG), 6, 53
diseases and disorders, 182–3; *see also under specific disorders*
Distillers Company (Biochemicals) Ltd, 9–11
division of labour in the family, 87, 93–4
Down's syndrome, 38, 82, 89, 146, 153, 158, 159, 162, 183
dryers, expenditure on, 112, 114, 115, 134
Du Boisson, M., 6
durable household goods, *see* consumer durables
Durkeim, E., 35
dwarfism (achondroplasia), 183

earnings, 72–94; loss of, 18, 23, 28, 49, 50, 54, 55, 56, 57, 73, 75–7, 82–3, 86, 88, 90–4, 95–6, 103–5, 135, 136, 138, 141, 155, 156, 164, 166, 170, 171, 172–3, 186; mens, 55, 66, 73, 85–94; women's, 55, 73–85
earnings-replacement benefit, 171, 172
employers, attitude of, 83, 87–8, 94
employment patterns of men, 85–94, 105–6; hours of work, 86, 87, 90–4, 141, 172; job changes, 86, 87, 105; job losses, 86, 87–8, 89–90; loss of promotion, 86, 88–9, 94, 105, 141, 185; overtime work, 87, 93; participation rates, 89–91; time off work, 87, 88, 94
employment patterns of women, 55, 73–85, 105; evening work, 81; hours of work, 75–7, 79, 81–4, 105; participation rates, 75; part-time work, 76–7, 81–3, 172; time off work, 77, 81, 82
Engels, F., 43
entertainment, expenditure on, 124, 125, 130, 145
epilepsy, 70, 90, 183
equipment, special, 132, 133, 189
expenditure, 51–63, 67, 107–40, 165, 166; overall, 128–32; *see also under specific commodities and services*
expenses allowance, 30, 171–2

Family Expenditure Survey (FES), 53, 61–8, 107–9, 176–82
Family Fund, 9–12, 24, 26, 27, 30, 55–6, 61–8, 114, 134, 167, 168, 170, 176–83
Family Fund Research Team, 26, 29, 55, 85, 182
family/state responsibilities, 40–5, 167
fares, *see* transport costs
food costs, 107, 108, 109–12, 128, 129, 130
footwear, expenditure on, *see* clothing and footwear costs
freezers, expenditure on, 124, 133
fuel costs, 107, 108, 112–15, 129, 130, 187
furniture, expenditure on, 124, 133, 134, 153–4, 189

General Household Survey (GHS), 53, 55
Goffman, E., 45

haemophilia, 183
Hall, P., 8, 9
Harris, A. I., 5, 7–8, 54
head injuries, 183
hearing, impaired, *see* deafness
heart disease, 82, 89, 120–1, 151, 183
heating costs, *see* fuel costs
Hewett, S., 55
hire purchase, *see* credit buying
Hodgkins disease, 183
holidays, 145, 146, 155
home-ownership, constraints on, 126, 151
hospital: costs associated with in-patient stays, 55, 107, 108, 132, 135–9, 156, 170, 190; costs associated with out-patient appointments, 135
housing costs (including adaptations), 87, 90, 107, 108, 126, 129, 132–3, 139, 149, 166, 170, 188–9
hydrocephalus, 183; *see also* spina bifida
Hyman, M., 56–7
hyperactivity, *see* behaviour problems

income, 53–9, 61–2, 66, 71–106, 165, 166; disposable, 101–4; from social security, 72, 94–106; gross, 71–101; relative to need, 102–3; sources of, 72
incontinence, 70, 81, 84, 114, 115, 117, 124, 131, 133, 134, 142, 143, 161, 184, 186–7

industrial injuries schemes, 7, 19–21, 23, 24, 173
institutional care, *see* residential care
insurance, life, 144, 148
invalid care allowance, 28, 172
Ison, T., 17

Jones, P., 22, 36–7
Joseph, Sir Keith, 11–12, 29
Joseph Rowntree Memorial Trust, 30
justice, social, 34–5

Kahn, A. J., 42
Kalton, G., 175
Kamerman, S. B., 42
Kew, S., 55
kidney failure, *see* renal failure
Kleinig, J., 48

Labour Party, 5
Labour Party Social Policy Committee, 5
Land, H., 42
life, rights to, 12, 38–40
lighting costs, *see* fuel costs
living standards, 51–2, 141–64, 165, 166, 170, 173
Living with Handicap (Younghusband Report), 10, 29
loans, 148–9, 170

McClements, L. D., 22
Maclean, M., 16
Marshall, T. H., 35
Martin, Jimmy, case of, 26
means tests, 159, 161, 168, 188
medicines, proprietary, expenditure on, 127
meningitis, 183
mental handicap, 12, 68, 70, 90, 109, 117, 152, 157, 158, 169, 183
microcephalus, 183
Mill, J. S., 43
miscellaneous goods, expenditure on, 108, 127–8, 129
'Misfortunes' survey, 54
mobility allowance, 24, 27–8, 30, 95–9, 102, 119–20, 122, 141, 154, 169, 171, 185
money management, *see* budgeting skills
mongolism, *see* Down's syndrome
Moroney, R. M., 41
Morris, A., 5

mortgages, *see* housing costs
muscular atrophy, 183
muscular dystrophy, 78, 183

National Health Service (Hospital Payments) Act (1973), 24
national insurance, 156, 157
need, concept of, 21, 35–6

occupational class, 64, 66–7, 89–93, 103–4, 179–82
Office of Population Censuses and Surveys (OPCS), 7, 53, 64, 175
opportunity costs, 49, 56

Parker, R., 42
Pearson Commission, *see* Royal Commission on Civil Liability and Compensation for Personal Injury
petrol costs, *see* transport costs
Piachaud, D., 55
Pigou, A. C., 46
Plant, R., 32
pressure groups, 4–7, 13, 54

rates, *see* housing costs
refrigerators, expenditure on, 124, 134
Registrar-General's classification of occupations, 66, 179–81
relatives, support from, 116, 142, 149
renal failure/disease, 136–8, 183
rent, *see* housing costs
Report on Compensation for Personal Injury in New Zealand (Woodhouse Report, 1972), 14
residential care, 41, 44–5
response rate, 64–5, 179
rheumatoid arthritis, *see* Still's disease
rights, *see* compensation, rights to; life, rights to; welfare, rights to; women's rights
Robens Committee on Safety and Health at work, 15
Royal Commission on Civil Liability and Compensation for Personal Injury (Pearson Commission), 2, 12, 14–15, 18, 24–7, 29–31, 99, 169, 171
Royal Commission on the Distribution of Income and Wealth, 53
rubella, maternal, 78, 164, 183

Safety and Health at Work Robens Committee Report), 15
Sainsbury, S., 5, 53, 54

sampling, 63–4, 66–8, 175–82
savings, personal, 144, 145, 148, 190
school, inability to attend, 170
school transport, 142–3
services (FES commodity group), expenditure on, 108, 124, 125–6, 129
services, for disabled children, 28–9, 166, 167; as opposed to cash benefits, 155, 160–4, 167, 168
severe disablement allowance, 173
shopping patterns, 110, 116, 143
skin complaints, 135, 152, 183
Social and Community Planning Research Ltd (SCPR), 64, 175
social class, *see* occupational class
Social Insurance and Allied Services (Beveridge Report, 1942), 20
social security: provision for disablement, 4, 6, 19–28; *see also* attendance allowance; cash benefits for disabled children; compensation; income, from social security; mobility allowance
Social Security Act (1973), 6, 8
Social Security Provision for Chronically Sick and Disabled People (House of Commons Paper, 276), 4, 8, 29
spina bifida, 12, 55, 68, 70, 81, 88, 110–11, 117, 138, 147, 150, 151, 155, 157, 159, 183
spina bifida and hydrocephalus, *see* spina bifida
standards of living, *see* living standards
Still's disease, 82, 114, 183
supplementary benefit, 7, 24, 102, 103

Tawney, R. H., 35
The Taxation of Husband and Wife (Cmnd. 8093), 172
taxis, expenditure on, *see* transport costs
telephones, expenditure on, 124, 125, 130, 133, 134, 188
television sets, expenditure on, 124, 133, 187
Thalidomide, 2, 5, 8–13, 15, 25, 29, 30, 47
Thornberry, B., 6
Titmuss, R. M., 22, 34, 36, 37, 46
tobacco costs, 108, 123–4, 129
toilet goods, expenditure on, 127, 131, 186
tort, 14, 16–23, 25
Townsend, P., 5, 15, 53
toys, expenditure on, 127, 136
transport costs, 59, 107, 108, 118–22, 129, 130, 131, 133, 134, 135, 136, 138, 149, 150, 163, 166, 169, 187
tuberose sclerosis, 183
tumours, 183

vaccine damage, 12, 24, 47, 173, 183
Vaccine Damage Payments Act (1979), 26
Voysey, M., 150

Walker, A., 15, 16, 35
war pensions schemes, 7, 20, 21, 23, 24
washing machines, use of and expenditure on, 112, 114, 124, 133–4, 189
welfare, rights to, 36–40, 46, 156–60, 167
Werdnig Hoffman disease (muscular atrophy), 183
wheelchairs, use of and expenditure on, 107, 115, 117, 118, 124, 134, 187, 189
women's rights, 43, 173
Woodburn, M. F., 55
Woodhouse Report (1972), 14
Workmen's Compensation Act (1897), 20

Younghusband Report (1970), 10, 29

For Product Safety Concerns and Information please contact our EU
representative GPSR@taylorandfrancis.com
Taylor & Francis Verlag GmbH, Kaufingerstraße 24, 80331 München, Germany

www.ingramcontent.com/pod-product-compliance
Lightning Source LLC
Chambersburg PA
CBHW061443300426
44114CB00014B/1818